FUNCTIONALLY ALERT BEHAVIOR
STRATEGIES

FAB

FUNCTIONALLY ALERT BEHAVIOR
STRATEGIES

INTEGRATED BEHAVIORAL, DEVELOPMENTAL, SENSORY, MINDFULNESS & MASSAGE TREATMENT

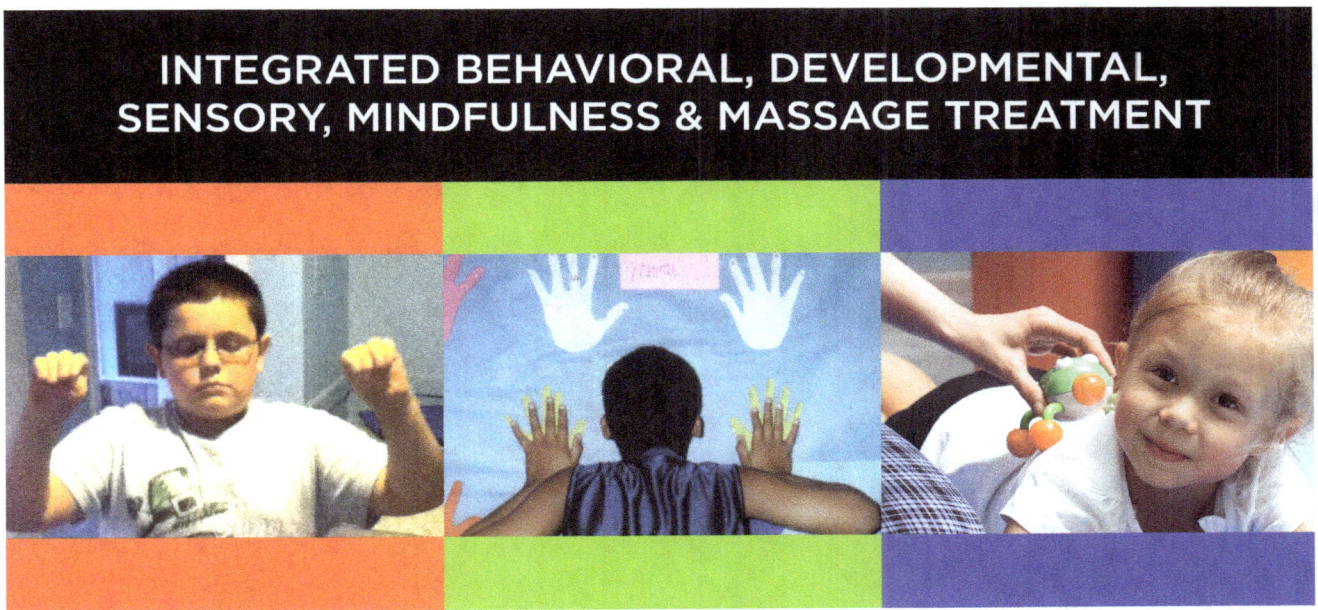

JOHN PAGANO, PH.D., OTR/L

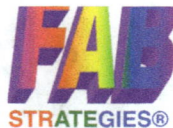

Copyrighted Material

FAB Functionally Alert Behavior Strategies: Integrated Behavioral, Developmental, Sensory, Mindfulness & Massage Treatment

Copyright © 2019 by Pagano FAB Strategies, LLC. All Rights Reserved.

No part of this publication may be reproduced, stored in a retrieval system or transmitted, in any form or by any means—electronic, mechanical, photocopying, recording or otherwise—without prior written permission from the publisher, except for the inclusion of brief quotations in a review.

For information about this title or to order other books and/or electronic media, contact the publisher:

Pagano FAB Strategies, LLC
Clinton, CT
www.fabstrategies.org
JLP96007@gmail.com

Library of Congress Preassigned Control Number: 2018913796

ISBNs
Softcover: 978-1-7328219-0-3
eBook: 978-1-7328219-1-0

Printed in the United States of America

Cover and Interior design: 1106 Design
Editor: Louise Bierig

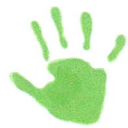

Dedicated to my son Patrick Pagano
and father Leonard Pagano

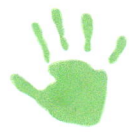

TABLE OF CONTENTS

Introducing FAB Strategies ix

Chapter 1 Environmental Adaptation Strategies 1

Chapter 2 Sensory Modulation Strategies 15

Chapter 3 FAB Pressure Touch Strategies 35

Chapter 4 Positive Behavior Support Strategies 49

Chapter 5 Physical Self-Regulation Strategies 65

Chapter 6 Individualizing Intervention with the FAB Strategies Form 77

Afterword: Expanding the Application of the FAB Strategies Curriculum 95

References 97

Index 105

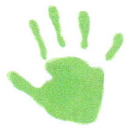

INTRODUCING FAB STRATEGIES

The FAB Strategies Approach

Many therapists, teachers, and parents struggle with students who don't pay attention, swear, tantrum, scream, hit, bite, or throw chairs. These complex behavioral challenges sabotage our ability to improve development, learning, and family life. It's impossible to effectively provide therapy, teach, or parent a student who is kicking you. FAB Strategies provide a practical, proven approach that simultaneously addresses inappropriate behavior as part of therapy, teaching, and parenting. It does not advocate trying the same approach with every student, but teaches a clinical reasoning approach of identifying the most important behavioral goal for a student and selecting the interventions that improve behavior.

Functionally Alert Behavior (FAB) Strategies are radical in their use of goal attainment in determining the therapy, teaching, and medical interventions to be used in coordinating these interventions. This provides the consistency necessary to embed treatment within the student's daily routine now and in the future. Practical methods are provided for quickly coordinating diverse interventions. On the basis of individualized assessment, strategies can be developed.

Evidence-based Clinical Reasoning and Therapeutic Intention

FAB Strategies apply the clinical reasoning process to improve a student's functional behavior. The clinical reasoning process involves therapists and teachers providing individualized consideration of current research evidence, the client's and family's values, the student's environment, objective progress toward functional behavioral goals, and possible risks.[1] By applying clinical reasoning,

FAB FUNCTIONALLY ALERT BEHAVIOR STRATEGIES

the therapist develops an individualized program integrating environmental adaptation, sensory modulation, positive behavior support, and physical self-regulation strategies. As a curriculum, FAB Strategies are applied individually to achieve each student's goal. The FAB Strategies form is used to guide clinical reasoning by selecting at least one strategy from each of the four categories: environmental adaptations, sensory modulation, positive behavior support, and physical self-regulation.

Therapeutic intention is the therapeutic use of self that conveys the true motivation of therapists and teachers in trying to modify a student's behavior. Although many therapists and teachers are unaware of their intentions, students with complex behavioral challenges intuitively understand and respond to them.

As an occupational therapist working with students who have complex behavioral challenges, I'm convinced that the intentions of therapists and teachers have a major impact on their effectiveness in improving behavior.[2] The radical uniqueness of occupational therapy's holistic perspective was best expressed by former American Occupational Therapy Association President Ginny Stoffel's statement that occupational therapy practitioners ask, "What matters to you?" not, "What's the matter with you?".[3]

Conveying genuine concern for their success is extremely important for improving behavior in students with complex behavioral challenges including developmental, sensory, intellectual, mental health, and post-traumatic stress disorders. Before students can trust therapists and teachers enough to change embedded behaviors, they have to be confident that the adults' intention is to help them have a better life. For this reason I have made it my lifelong effort to uncover and purify my intentions as a therapist, teacher, workshop leader, and author.

In this introduction I want to share the personal and professional experiences that have shaped my intentions. Like many people in the helping professions, my professional choices were influenced by personal experience. When I was a young child, my beloved sister was born with Down syndrome. Although my mother knew immediately that something was different with her third child, the pediatrician said my sister was "fine and would grow out of her differences." When my sister died of pneumonia as a toddler and my mother read "Down syndrome" on her death certificate, my family felt betrayed by the medical profession; however, the truth gave us peace.

Individuals with Down syndrome have distinctive facial features and physical characteristics. As a fourteen-year-old, I found them frightening. I felt ashamed of my reaction and decided I would confront my fears by going to the Central Connecticut Regional Center down the street from where I lived and registering as a volunteer to work with "handicapped" children. I still remember my first experience when an overwhelmed childcare worker told me to sit down and placed a crying child with cerebral palsy on my lap before she hurried off to comfort another client.

As the child immediately relaxed in my arms and stopped crying, I lost my fear of the "developmentally disabled" and saw these kids as individuals with challenges and joys just like everyone else. I volunteered frequently at the regional center, discovering that I liked and had a gift for working with children who had complex developmental challenges. When I turned sixteen, I was hired part-time at the regional center as a recreational therapist.

When considering a career, I admired the work of the physical therapists at the regional center but was drawn to working with the occupational therapists. At that time occupational therapy (OT) was a relatively new mind and body therapy, mainly teaching kids with disabilities such things as how to feed and dress themselves. Occupational therapy emphasized living fully by engaging in meaningful activities that promote integrated healing of the mind, body, and spirit.

In college I chose occupational therapy as a major, and it felt right to me. This was in 1977, and at the time the concept in OT of an integrated mind, body, and spirit was considered a bit radical, but now it's just something that "everyone always knew." I got my BS degree and license in OT and began working with children, adolescents, and young adults who had developmental disabilities. Over the years I've continued working with youth who have developmental disabilities, but I became increasingly focused on the behavioral challenges that seemed to most greatly limit them functionally.

Professional distance was emphasized in college, but an early professional experience convinced me of the importance of maintaining a caring attitude toward all of the individuals I served. I was working as an occupational therapist in a pediatric intensive care unit, and I was deeply affected by my work with a particular infant who was born prematurely and addicted to drugs. I was asked to work extensively with the infant because he had severe pulmonary distress that the nurses noticed was improved when I held, cared for, and massaged him.

Although it was clear to everyone that he would eventually die, the doctors worked diligently to save him, reviving him countless times before assessing that he was "brain dead" and should be allowed to die painlessly. When he died I was devastated, but I felt that the love and care of the medical staff hadn't been wasted. I was touched by a spiritual experience conveying to me that this child's life had had great significance. I felt compelled to express the importance of relationships in the poem "Intensive Caring."

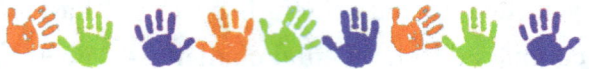

Intensive Caring

The waves of your heartbeats
Float waves across the screen
Amidst all the machinery
You barely can be seen
Fragile, frightened little boy
With cries so faint yet shrill
There's no one here to hold you tight
So, little boy, I will.

Recalling myself as a troubled youth
Reveals to me a startling truth
I know so well why my heart cries
Out to the little boy who tries.

For me our journey has defined
The ways our struggles are entwined
Like the leads that from the start
Monitored your tiny heart
And yet no monitor perceives
The hands that give also receive
I hope my hands transmit the joy
You've brought to our lives, little boy.

Doctors dance to the tune of the monitor chimes
Chanting children pay for societal crimes
Jesus whispers, *John, look beyond the disease
My kingdom belongs to such as these.*

The last time I saw my fragile friend
I knew his life had reached its end

INTRODUCING FAB STRATEGIES

The nurse who most loved him shrilly cried
Our little angel now had died.

I saw his body lying there
And felt much pain, but no despair
He gave so very much to me
Did I learn what he wanted me to see?
He got me to ask what it means to care
For another to be truly there
His shrouded body reveals a truth that is real
When we give of our whole selves, we truly heal.

Doctors dance to the tune of the monitor chimes
Chanting children pay for societal crimes
Jesus whispers, *John, look beyond the disease*
My kingdom belongs to such as these.

Expanding My Training by Filling in the Gaps

As an occupational therapist, I find that my training in using meaningful activities, play, swings, sensory integration, massage, scrub brushing, Trager bodywork, massage, and Brain Gym activities works. These methods integrate well with the special education and family therapy approaches I learned in graduate school. These interventions motivate youngsters with complex behavioral challenges. As a proud pediatric occupational therapist, I am still occasionally criticized by some pediatricians and behaviorists for my "OT voodoo practices" of play, massage, and sensory-based interventions. This criticism used to bother me; but after thirty-five years working with clients who have complex behavioral challenges, my evidence-based practices and my clients' functional improvements make these interventions a source of pride.

Occupational therapists are gifted professionals, and I'm proud to be one of them. However, my knowledge after graduating lacked a holistic view of children, so I went back to college part-time to get a multidisciplinary MS degree in Early Childhood Special Education. My MS coursework involved studying early childhood education, special education, counseling, and speech/language pathology. I learned much in my training with diverse teachers and allied health professionals.

When addressing complex behavioral challenges, the health care professions often seem like an orchestra comprised of competing sections trying to drown each other out. While the various professionals have a responsibility to focus on the client's medical, physical, occupational, communication, or educational needs, they also need to recognize that they are treating a unified individual.

Students with complex developmental challenges come to therapists as a whole individual and then are directed to a physical therapist to help them learn to walk, an occupational therapist to improve their functional fine motor skills, a speech/language pathologist to teach them to talk, and mental health therapists to reduce their feelings of sadness and improve their behavior. As a "birth-to-three" occupational therapist, I was suddenly directed to be a transdisciplinary therapist who addressed all the needs of the infant and family, including helping some parents with severe financial and substance abuse challenges. In many ways I felt a spiritual calling to get my doctoral degree even though I had no real need for one as an occupational therapist. I just felt drawn to a greater understanding of the families that so strongly supported the children I served, so I enrolled part-time in the University of Connecticut Marriage and Family Therapy program, where I eventually obtained my PhD.

My doctoral studies and dissertation reinforced the importance of using a transdisciplinary process that includes caring about the infant and family to maximize an infant's developmental progress. My dissertation focused on the impact of therapy on parental stress, a factor that significantly affects children's development. In my doctoral research, I studied the impact of feeding intervention by birth-to-three occupational and speech/language therapists on parental stress. To my surprise,

INTRODUCING FAB STRATEGIES

receipt of feeding therapy both positively and negatively affected parental stress, and whether the feeding interventions were successful or not did not affect that stress. Instead, my quantitative and qualitative research indicated that parental stress was significantly reduced if parents felt that their child's therapist cared about and valued them and their child as individuals. In contrast, parental stress increased if the parent felt that their child's therapist did not think the parent was doing enough for their child.[4]

Even more surprising to me, when piloting my dissertation, was noticing that parents often perceived that their therapist felt that they as parents were not doing enough for their infant because they were unable to complete the therapist's extensive home feeding programs. Parents expressed the importance of having therapists ask more about their home life so they could embed home programs into their daily routine. Parents suggested that this could be done by, for example, advising them to provide input to the mouth during bathing, when the parent already had to be with their toddler because they needed to provide individual attention during bathing to ensure their toddler wouldn't drown. This advice helps me be realistic when providing home program suggestions and to embed home interventions into a family's daily routine.

In addition to learning the importance of caring, I was taught the necessity of self-care and balance by recognizing the extreme stress that comes with working with students who have complex behavioral challenges. In addition to an hour of daily exercise, I practice centering prayer[5] a half hour each day. Centering prayer is a Christian mindfulness practice that reduces a practitioner's anxiety while enhancing their sense of Christian spiritual growth.[6] It is important to practice mindfulness regularly in order to effectively teach it to students. Research indicates that mindfulness practice decreases stress and improves the effectiveness of therapists, teachers, and parents who have children with complex behavioral challenges.

For me, practicing regular centering prayer thirty minutes daily and once weekly in a group reduces my stress and improves my intention as a therapist. Teachers and therapists can explore various mindfulness practices and find a group and daily time to practice the one they like best. In addition to this daily practice, I do the 4–4–6–2 breath-counting strategy (described in Chapter 2 Sensory Modulation Strategies) to gain self-control in moments of extreme stress.

I have been working in my current job at an adolescent psychiatric hospital for ten years. When I arrived, all of the hospital staff—from the superintendent to the childcare workers—was motivated to reduce, and if possible, eliminate the use of restraint and seclusion. My impression was that the practice of touching and giving attention to clients only when they were violent was reinforcing their aggression. Hospital-wide policies were changed to include staff-supported use of massage, adaptive equipment, and a client-centered approach to empowering clients to find coping strategies to replace their aggressive behaviors. As a result of the hospital staff's comprehensive efforts, we were able to eliminate the use of restraint beds and locked seclusion rooms.[7]

FAB FUNCTIONALLY ALERT BEHAVIOR STRATEGIES

Applying FAB Strategies and Using the FAB Strategies Form

The FAB Strategies presented in this book were developed through extensive research and thirty-one years of clinical trial with students who have complex behavioral challenges. FAB Strategies were refined through my experience teaching them in workshops over the past twenty-one years to preschool and kindergarten teachers, as well as to occupational, speech/language, physical, and mental health therapists. FAB Strategies are a practical, evidence-based, multidisciplinary approach for therapists and teachers working with students who have complex behavioral challenges.

The FAB Strategies described in this book are unique in their integration of behavioral and sensory strategies. Some therapists and teachers attending FAB Strategies trainings are surprised by the combination of both research-supported behavioral strategies and fun sensory strategies for use with students who have complex behavioral challenges. This dual emphasis was developed through my thirty-five years as an occupational therapist. When working with students who have complex behavioral challenges, it is important that therapists use the most effective research-based interventions and present them through an individualized approach so students will do them. FAB Strategies also differ from traditional behavioral and sensory strategies in that they provide a curriculum of practical, evidence-based interventions that therapists and teachers can use to develop individualized interventions.

Although little research has been done on integrating developmental, behavioral, sensory, mindfulness, and massage strategies, this approach has been used extensively in clinical practice with students who have complex behavioral challenges. Research tends to address a specific treatment for a single distinct diagnosis such as autism, whereas clinicians often treat students who have complex behavioral challenges and multiple diagnoses of post-traumatic stress disorder, intellectual disability, autism spectrum disorder, and schizophrenia; these students require combined interventions.

The extreme importance of individualized inclusion of developmental, behavioral, sensory, mindfulness, and massage interventions for some students with complex behavioral challenges is that integrating these strategies best addresses their behavioral challenges. While behaviorism has been proven for autism spectrum disorder alone, it may need to be integrated with other approaches if the student also has post-traumatic stress disorder, an intellectual disability, and significant sensory modulation difficulties. Sensory strategies seem to be helpful for many pediatric psychiatric disorders because they reduce anxiety and aggression.

The FAB Strategies form guides individualization of the curriculum to help achieve the student's most important initial goal (see Figure I.1). Interventions listed on the FAB Strategies form are designated in boldface in this book, whereas suggested strategies not listed on the form are indicated in boldface italic type. Two lines are set at the bottom of the FAB Strategies form; there, therapists can list any of the italicized FAB Pre-K and Kindergarten or additional strategies they want to include.

INTRODUCING FAB STRATEGIES

It is important to choose the most important initial goal to address. The FAB Strategies form provides strategies presented in four sections: environmental adaptation, sensory modulation, positive behavior support, and physical self-regulation. The form is individualized to achieve the functional behavioral goals specified on the top of the form.

The FAB Strategies form is a useful checklist for remembering effective strategies for students with complex behavioral challenges. It can be used while planning treatment and during individual sessions to record useful strategies and plan strategies to try during the next treatment session. It is also useful for providing home program strategies that can be shared with the student's family, teachers, and other therapists. Teams will also find the form to be useful because it allows all the teachers and therapists working with a student to provide interventions in a consistent way.[8]

Pertinent details about the student and their therapy are written in the blanks at the top of the form. The form includes four sections: environmental adaptation, sensory modulation, positive behavior support, and physical self-regulation. When individualizing the form for a student, interventions are selected by checking the line to the left, then selecting strategies in that row by underlining them. Beneath the last strategy are two rows for adding applicable strategies that are not already listed. Below these lines are a list of websites that can be referred to and a list of references. A parent or guardian signs the bottom of the form, indicating that they support the program.

FAB FUNCTIONALLY ALERT BEHAVIOR STRATEGIES

Figure I.1 FAB Strategies to Improve Self-Control Form

Copyright © 2019 by John Pagano, Ph.D., OTR/L, www.fabstrategies.org
Permission granted for direct use with clients.

X: therapist   √: family/teacher   A: Attachment

Client: _____ Therapist: _____ Contact: _____
Functional Goals: _____ Dates: _____

A. ENVIRONMENTAL ADAPTATION
____ Sensory coping area/Prepare-Limit-Transitions/Low noise/Headphones/Fidget-Comfort Box-Bag
____ **Ear Press/Weighted-Blanket-Pressure-Vest/Pencil grip/Chewy/Sit: Stable-Separate-Carrel-Disk**
____ Visual: List-Schedule-If then/Schedule story/Sit near teacher/Calm face/Slow: Speech-Pace
____ Choice of 1 activity from . . . 4 choices; do ____ minutes minimum; clean up before next activity

B. SENSORY MODULATION
____ Arousal level-Modulate/Coping strategies/Breathing: Hand-Bird-4462/Mindful clock: Sit-Stand
____ Freeze dance/Giant steps/Simon says/Deliver: Books-Messages-Box/Rolling to Read-Math
____ Beans & Rice-Theraputty-Sand-Playdoh-Water-Glue-Shaving cream/Self-brushing
____ Vibration/Back: X-Crawl/Tap-Press self: Fingers to ear-Head to feet/Roll therapy ball-Core
____ **Touch: Back-Arm/Head crown/Shoulders: Squeeze-Press/Spine roll/Back tech: Tap-Press**
____ **Supported sitting therapy ball: Forward & back-Up & down-Sides-Mindful clock**

C. POSITIVE BEHAVIOR SUPPORT
____ Ask permission to kid-Touch/Prompt filter speech/Invite/Will like you/Social role-play/Redirect
____ Breaks/Self-management/Tolerance for delay/Conditioned calm recall/Sensory matching
____ Pre-correction/Practice saying/Coping card/FAB Turtle/Humor/Desensitization/Partial sentences
____ Preferred: Tasks-Distractor/Choices/Break-Mand/Intersperse learned tasks/Priming/Prompts
____ Reinforce: Attempts-Appropriate-Point chart-Tangible/Desensitization/Self-management

D. PHYSICAL SELF-REGULATION
____ Push wall/Push-ups-Wall/Exercise band activities/Cardio machines/Weight lift/Punch heavy bag
____ Prone on therapy ball: Hands rock-Wheelbarrow walk/Mini-trampoline jump/Play structure
____ Flex & extend shoulder & ankle: Same-Opposite-Opposite, adding shoulder halfway up & down
____ Both-Hand: Same-side knee-*Eyes down right*/Opposite knee-*Eyes up left*
____ Diagonal-X-Infinity I-Alternate I-I visually track/Pre-check twist/Elbow I/Symmetry
____ Ball: Wall-Letter-Quadruped pass-Bat-Bounce activities/Beanbag pass activities
____ **Crash Pad/Scooter board: Pull-Push/Suspended Swing: Forward-Back-Lateral-Spin-Target**
____ Activities: _____
____ Activities: _____

www.fabstrategies.org   www.challengingbehavior.org   www.spdstar.org
References: Domitrovich et al., 2013; Koester, 2012; LaVigna & Willis, 2012; Stahmer et al., 2011

Parent/Guardian Signature Supporting Program: _____

Developing FAB Strategies

The FAB Strategies taught in this book have evolved over the twenty-one years I've been teaching them, and they continue to do so. At this point they comprise a multidisciplinary curriculum for children, adolescents, and young adults who have complex behavioral challenges.

FAB Strategies focus on improving functional behavior. Functional behavior is an important determinant of success that our fragmented medical, allied health, and school systems inadequately address. Occupational, physical, speech/language, and mental health therapists are trained to be one integral part of a multidisciplinary team working to achieve the client's functional goals.

The team working to help youth with complex behavioral challenges includes parents, teachers, behaviorists, pediatricians, pediatric psychiatrists, neurologists, and occupational, physical, speech/language, mental health, music, and art therapists. All team members need to work together to help these youth, who often have developmental, mental health, and sensory problems in addition to complex behavioral challenges. I invite you to join me in using and developing FAB Strategies.

CHAPTER 1

ENVIRONMENTAL ADAPTATION STRATEGIES

Environmental adaptation strategies provide an evidence-based foundation for intervention with students who have complex behavioral challenges. Useful environmental adaptation strategies can include adaptive equipment, visual supports, and adaptive sensory techniques. These are distinct from the more common practice of randomly using adaptive equipment, toys, and techniques. Environmental adaptation strategies are most effective when individualized to improve goal-directed behavior. All of a student's therapists and teachers need to use environmental adaptations consistently.

Although often minimized and given insufficient attention, individualized environmental adaptations should be the first consideration for preventing, rather than reacting to, inappropriate behavior. Environmental adaptations are a universal-level positive behavioral support that reduces anxiety and promotes positive behavior in all students. All programs to support positive behavior stress the importance of a structured classroom environment that minimizes noise and visual distractions, particularly for students with complex behavioral challenges.

In these students, individualized environmental adaptations are particularly helpful for minimizing stress and promoting attention for learning. Environmental adaptations to improve behavior are most effective when introduced one at a time as an experiment. They are continued if the adaptation is used appropriately and results in progress toward behavioral goal attainment. These adaptations can also be used strategically as motivation and reinforcement for appropriate behavior in school. Section A of the FAB Strategies form, environmental adaptations, lists helpful adaptive equipment, visual support, and basic organizational strategies that can be individualized to improve behavior (see Figure I.1).

Guidelines for Using Adaptive Equipment

Specifying the guidelines for continued use before giving students adaptive equipment (e.g., allowing students to chew gum or use fidget toys in class) avoids potential problems and ensures that any long-term environmental adaptations are used to promote goal attainment. Many teachers dislike environmental adaptations because they interfere with classroom management or don't help improve behavior (e.g., chewing gum is problematic because students stick their gum on the chairs after use; fidget toys cause disruptions because students throw or make loud noises with them). Establishing clear rules for continued use, behavioral goals, and baseline data makes teachers and principals more eager to encourage the use of adaptive equipment.

If specific adaptive equipment is not significantly reducing problematic behavior, its use needs to be reconsidered. Behavioral problems can be worsened by the inappropriate use of adaptive equipment and sensory strategies, so it is important to assess severe behavioral problems before introducing adaptive equipment or sensory strategies. Once adaptive equipment is chosen, it should be introduced in a manner that will maximize success.

Given current school inclusion practices, many classes have students with diverse developmental levels. To help all students, teachers and therapists should initially explain to the class that everyone has different needs and abilities, and each student will be treated "fairly" but not "equally." Students are given different rules, equipment, and expectations based on their individual needs. The students then try the adaptive equipment "for the day as an experiment that will be continued only if used appropriately to help reach your goal."

It is important to select adaptive equipment that the student likes and wants to use. In using desired adaptive equipment, students are reinforced for working toward their goals, and they are awarded a sticker or other pre-specified reinforcement for making progress. After trying the adaptive equipment and recording goal progress for two weeks, it can be determined whether the environmental adaptation should be continued, modified, or discontinued.

An important guideline is to balance environmental structure through adaptive equipment before increasing demands; for example, provide noise-canceling headphones to block out audible distractions before introducing academically challenging learning activities. Reducing behavioral demands is helpful in less-structured environments. When clients first begin showing anxiety or behavioral difficulties, assess how the environmental supports match the demands being made, and adjust the environmental adaptations accordingly.

Adaptive equipment can be useful in reducing sensory distractions. Academic achievement and behavior can be enhanced in students with anxiety, limited attention, and sensory hyper-reactivity by simultaneously reducing auditory, visual, and tactile distractions. Useful classroom adaptations include sound-absorbing walls, noise-canceling headphones, carpeting to reduce audible distractions, and halogen lighting and study carrels to minimize extraneous visual stimuli.[1] Specific seating away from peers can help to promote attention in students with sensory over-responsivity by eliminating the competing sensory stimuli of accidentally touching peers while listening to or looking at the teacher.

In addition to reducing distractions, adaptive equipment can be used to add sensory input that enhances learning. *Color highlighting print* and *adding manipulative activities* such as blocks when counting or tactile letters when learning the alphabet can highlight learning cues for students with sensory oversensitivity and attention deficit hyperactivity disorder (ADHD). Focus can be enhanced for some students by having them simultaneously read and listen to a story. An *audiovisual (AV) system* can be particularly useful for students with auditory processing problems by increasing the volume of the teacher's voice so it is louder than competing stimuli. These sensory strategies can promote learning better than ADHD medication for some students.[2]

Environmental Adaptation Strategies

The environmental adaptation strategies from section A of the FAB Strategies form are described in order below. Items from the FAB Strategies form are set in boldface, FAB Strategies from the pre-K and kindergarten form as well as strategies not on the form that can be added on the activity lines at the bottom are set in italics.

The **sensory coping area** is a designated area students can use to avoid misbehavior when they or their teacher notice they are experiencing environmental or body triggers. For example, a student can be guided to identify that being told "no" is their greatest environmental trigger, whereas acting mean is their body trigger, before becoming aggressive. As soon as a therapist calls attention to these triggers, the student is encouraged to do push-ups, his preferred and most effective coping strategy. Sensory coping areas help students modulate their arousal level and reduce the need for seclusion. Students are reinforced for using the area to avoid inappropriate behavior.

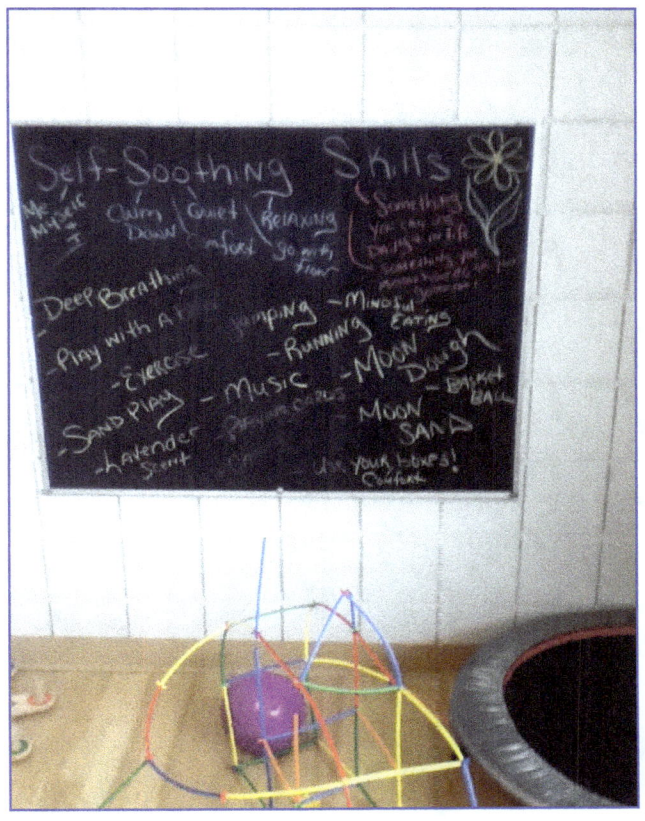

Teachers and therapists can design sensory coping areas to meet classroom needs. This may be a designated seat and desk with masking tape on the floor marking the boundaries for students to use, with the teacher's permission, rather than working at their assigned desk. For students with significant developmental, behavioral, and sensory modulation challenges, the sensory coping area might be a pup tent with mats and cushions that limit sensory input and provide deep-pressure input.

FAB FUNCTIONALLY ALERT BEHAVIOR STRATEGIES

In some schools, group homes, psychiatric residential units, and juvenile detention facilities, a *sensory coping room* is helpful. This is a separate room, distinct from a punitive break or time-out room, where youth voluntarily choose to go to calm down. It can be useful to initially assess environmental adaptations in the sensory coping room, or to suggest students go there when they are upset to avoid aggression toward themselves or others. Use of a sensory coping area can significantly reduce distress in adolescents with psychiatric illness.[3]

The FAB Sensory Coping Room Log objectively assesses the usefulness of a sensory coping area or room and helps determine the most effective sensory coping area interventions (see Figure 1.1). When used as components of a comprehensive program, the Sensory Coping Room Log and a sensory coping room significantly reduced patient distress and restraint in an adolescent psychiatric hospital.[4] The FAB Sensory Coping Room Log provides objective data regarding the effectiveness of using the area or room and which coping strategies are most effective.

ENVIRONMENTAL ADAPTATION STRATEGIES

Figure 1.1. FAB SENSORY COPING ROOM LOG

Copyright © 2019 by John Pagano, Ph.D., OTR/L www.fabstrategies.org
Permission granted to copy for individual clinical use

Child: _____ Staff: _____
Date: _____ Time: _____ Sensory Coping Room use suggested by: Child: _____ Staff: _____

CIRCLE ENTERING LEVEL OF UPSET

1	2	3	4	5	6	7	8	9	10
CALM				Medium			Angry		AGGRESSIVE

Behavior before sensory coping room use: _____

ENVIRONMENT (CHECK ITEMS USED)
Dim lighting _____ *Pup tent* _____ *Noise-canceling headphones* _____
Weighted blanket _____ *Weighted vest* _____ *Weighted shawl* _____
Bean Bag Chair _____ *Music* _____ *Programs/CDs* _____ *Lycra pressure vest* _____
Rocking Chair _____ *Body sock* _____ *Aromatherapy* _____ *Scent* _____
Other _____

ACTIVITIES (CHECK ITEMS USED)
_____ *Decrease then gradually increase sensory input/Increase structure/Speak slow/Calm face*
_____ *Stretch: Up-Side-Twist-Down-Forward*
_____ *Nose breathe out: double in fist thumb-Tense & relax*
_____ *Push-ups: Wall-Knee-Marine wall-Regular*
_____ *TheraBand-Exercise tubing: Forward, Down, Cross Midline*
_____ *Self-brushing-Isometrics: Up & Down-Center-Down*
_____ *Talk with staff-Specific peer-Telephone family*
_____ *Steamroller Deluxe time in up to:* _____
_____ *Favorite Toys Type* _____
_____ *Therapy putty-Wiki Stix-Crafts Type:* _____
_____ *Fidget-Vibrating toys Type:* _____
_____ *Therapy ball: Bounce seated-Push-ups-Rock on hands-Wheelbarrow walk*
_____ *Chewy Type* _____
_____ *Mini-trampoline jumping-Punch heavy bag*
Other _____

CIRCLE LEVEL OF UPSET AFTER USE

1	2	3	4	5	6	7	8	9	10
CALM				Medium			Angry		AGGRESSIVE

Behavior after sensory coping room use: _____

Prepare transitions involves previewing upcoming transitions to assist with the frustration tolerance involved in going from one activity to the next. A warning five and two minutes before transitions helps students prepare for transitions. Music, chimes, or other auditory signals can be useful before and during a transition to help designate the time before quitting one activity and starting the next. Boardmaker software offers an easy way to quickly develop individualized picture schedules that can be posted to help make students aware of upcoming transitions.

Transitions require students to alternate from one set of sensory inputs to another and can be made more predictable through the use of consistent visual or written schedules. Whenever possible, buffer activities can be used to limit the need for children to go from highly favorable to unfavorable activities. For example, if a preschool class needs to come in from the playground and transition to naptime, a buffer activity such as snack and stretching helps the transition from active to relaxed time and prevents the need for the children to transition directly from a highly preferred activity to a much less favorable activity.

Limit transitions help clients with sensory modulation or behavioral flexibility challenges benefit behaviorally by reducing the number of transitions that need to occur. This technique can be extremely effective when used in conjunction with the prepare transitions strategy. Alternating between activities is a common environmental trigger, especially for young and developmentally challenged children.

Physical Strategies

Low noise involves keeping the noise volume within the class or home setting low. Attention is given to environmental adaptations such as carpeting that reduce noise levels, and if needed, the use of noise-canceling headphones. Students tend to behave better when the noise level of the room is kept low.

Headphones refer to noise-canceling headphones to reduce noise levels that negatively affect distractibility or behavior. Headphones can reduce distress by blocking out extraneous noise such as fire alarms.[5] A related evidence-based strategy shown to improve learning and reduce anxiety in students with developmental disabilities is the use of *room carpeting* and *sound-absorbing walls* to reduce noise distractions.

A **fidget** is a manipulative or textured toy that provides sensory tactile input so children don't touch others and are better able to pay attention. Fidgets and other adaptive equipment can be placed in a **comfort box**, a shoebox decorated with the student's name and behavioral goal on it. Fidgets and other manipulative objects can be gradually added to the comfort box as the students increasingly demonstrate appropriate use of the objects and progress toward their goals.

ENVIRONMENTAL ADAPTATION STRATEGIES

A **comfort bag** is filled with manipulative adaptive equipment and favorite toys or electronic gadgets (e.g., Nintendo, Candy Crush Saga game) that are only offered during high-stress times that require waiting or other high demands (e.g., haircuts, doctor's appointments, shopping). The child has access to the **comfort bag** as long as all the rules are followed, but if they misbehave, all items are returned to the comfort bag, and the appointment is canceled.

Strategies Conducted by a Therapist

The next eleven strategies set in boldface are to be conducted by or under the direction of an occupational, physical, or speech/language therapist trained in sensory behavioral strategies.

The **ear press strategy** is useful for clients who may benefit from noise-canceling or therapeutic-listening headphones but refuse to try them. Many clients who are hyper-responsive to sound are also oversensitive to touch and reluctant to try noise-canceling or auditory integration headphones because they are bothered by wearing something over their ears. The **ear press strategy** involves describing then providing, through touch, deep pressure on both ears for ten seconds, followed by having the student voluntarily wear noise-canceling headphones for progressively longer periods to earn a reward. Individuals with hyper-responsivity to sound are frequently hypersensitive to touch as well and so will refuse to try using headphones to block sound because they feel uncomfortable. The deep pressure and initial reinforcement can be useful to minimize irritation from the touch input of the headphones, enabling the use of headphones in reducing auditory distractibility. An alternative for students who really dislike the touch from the headphones is to provide them for use in fire drills and other times of extremely loud noise.

A **weighted blanket** can be useful for calming students, particularly those with a history of post-traumatic stress disorder. Use of a **weighted blanket** weighing thirty pounds significantly decreases distress and arousal levels in adults. Trials of the weighted blanket in the sensory coping area can be especially helpful in initially determining its effectiveness as a coping strategy. Research also supports the effectiveness of individualized use of the **weighted vest** for improving attention in students with ADHD. Weighted vests and weighted blankets are calming for some students with developmental disabilities, and wearing time is often limited only by preference and the inability to breathe comfortably.

The **weighted vest** is traditionally a maximum of 10 percent of body weight and is worn for up to forty-five minutes, followed by forty-five minutes with the vest off; but therapists may choose to try greater weight and durations. Weighted vests can be helpful if used individually for students with ADHD to improve attention, on-task behavior,[6] and in-seat behavior.[7] Research indicates that weighted vests are not effective for decreasing repetitive behaviors in youth with autism spectrum disorder.[8] The greatest contraindication for using weighted vests and weighted blankets is chest compression, particularly in clients with neuromuscular or respiratory problems. This issue must be closely monitored; have the therapist watch while the client wears the weighted blanket and remove it immediately if the client dislikes the experience or begins to have any difficulty breathing. An occupational therapist should determine the use of a weighted vest on an individual basis, by assuring that post-test use improves functioning by being repeatedly found to increase attention or decrease distress.[9]

A **pressure vest** can help reduce anxiety and improve attention. Pressure vests are often tried before a weighted vest because they are more discrete and thus have the practical advantage of eliminating stigma for students. Pressure vests are available commercially and can be worn under clothes or with spandex outerwear, sports shirts, and vests for students who don't want to "look different." The spandex can also be sewn into custom shirts and vests.

Pressure shorts are an alternative included on the FAB Strategies Pre-K & Kindergarten form that can be added to the bottom of the FAB Strategies form for students who masturbate in public. For these students, bike shorts or one-piece wrestling singlets can be worn as an environmental barrier and sensory strategy. Students can simultaneously be given reinforcement for going progressively longer periods without inappropriately touching themselves.

A **pencil grip** is the use of various types of pencil grip attachments to improve writing ease or legibility. Pencil grips are commercially available or can be individualized by using splinting material or customized 3-D printing. It is important to try the pencil grip and ensure that it consistently makes writing easier or more legible.

A **chewy** is a **sensory matching strategy** that can be useful as nonsocial automatic reinforcement for students with inappropriate mouthing behavior (e.g., hand mouthing, pica, biting, sleeve sucking). It is best for an occupational and behavioral therapist to develop this type of replacement strategy collaboratively. For example, if students are causing skin abrasions by repeatedly mouthing their fingers, the therapists may assume that water play and use of a chewy will more appropriately provide the nonsocial automatic sensory input the student is seeking through finger sucking. This sensory matching strategy is supported by research as non-contingent reinforcement with a matched sensory input.[10] The children are allowed to use a chewy and water play whenever they want and are simultaneously rewarded for going progressively longer periods without mouthing their fingers.

Sitting Strategies

Sit stable involves modifying the height and length of a chair to a student's size so they are in an optimally stable sitting position while listening to the teacher and doing their schoolwork. For students with postural balance difficulties and fear of falling, optimally stable sitting can help them feel

ENVIRONMENTAL ADAPTATION STRATEGIES

secure and able to concentrate. According to the "automaticity deficit framework" hypothesis, some children need to concentrate to maintain upright sitting and they lack adequate postural stability for optimal proficiency in fine motor activities, or the effort to remain upright distracts them from attending.[11] Optimally stable sitting ensures that children are upright and symmetrical, with the chair supporting their pelvis at approximately a 90-degree angle. The hips and knees are also flexed at 90-degree angles such that they are straight, with the ankles also flexed approximately 90 degrees so that the feet are flat on the floor.

Sit separate involves placing a student's desk at a distance far enough away from those next to him so that he will not accidentally be touched or talked to by others. Often masking tape, stop signs, and other visual supports can help maintain the separateness of the seating area. Students with tactile defensiveness and sensory oversensitivity attend best when they are not simultaneously exposed to touch and sound. Because students with autism spectrum disorder and sensory over-responsivity have significantly decreased neural habituation, the sit separate strategy can help improve their behavior by keeping them from being overwhelmed by repeated simultaneous auditory and tactile stimulation in class.[12]

Sit carrel is the use of a study carrel or a poster board placed on or between desks to help direct students' attention to their own work by reducing visual distractions.[13] This is particularly helpful for mainstreamed students who have a one-to-one assistant and need to visually attend to their desktop in a noisy room with lots of movement. Students with a history of sensory modulation or post-traumatic stress disorder (PTSD) often are hyper-vigilant to those around them and benefit from directing their attention to the work on their desktop.

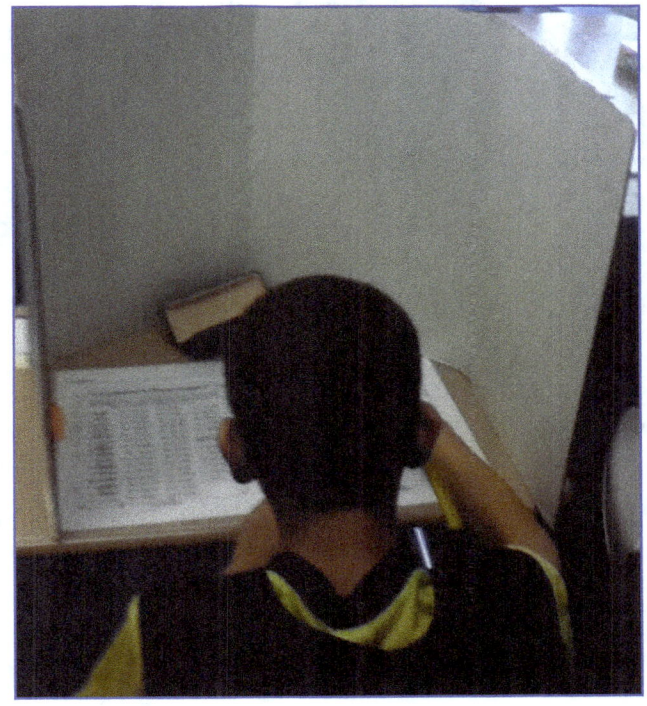

A *slant board* is a related option that frequently helps promote visual attention to classwork. It is a downward-slanted board that can include a *clipboard* attachment. The *slant board* can promote visual processing during reading and writing as well as facilitate an upright rather than hunched posture. A clipboard can be useful during challenging writing assignments for students who have difficulty stabilizing their paper while writing. *Halogen lighting* is another evidence-based strategy that reduces visual distractions and enhances learning for students with developmental disabilities.

FAB FUNCTIONALLY ALERT BEHAVIOR STRATEGIES

Assigned seats is an extremely useful strategy for preschoolers and kindergarteners that strategically place students near peers who will best reduce distraction and conflicts and best promote learning.[14] In addition to placing students who don't get along far away from each other, therapists and teachers can seat students with developmental delays next to peers with slightly better developmental skills to serve as optimal language or behavioral models.

The *tray* and **carpet square** strategy provides physical barriers to define personal boundaries. Every student is assigned a tray for his or her work materials and a carpet square for assigned floor seating. Students are rewarded for using only the materials on their tray and staying seated on their carpet square, with consequences for touching other students' tray or carpet square "bubbles" without permission. Trays and carpet squares can be individualized or kept consistent to avoid conflicts over receiving the "best" items.

The **sit disk** is an effective initial strategy for increasing in-seat attention by letting the student sit on a Disc-o-Sit, a commercially available inflated seat cushion that provides texture and encourages movement. For students who are still unable to remain seated using a sit disk, additional strategies to encourage seated attention include *sit with TheraBand or exercise tubing tied to the chair handle or legs, sit on a therapy ball within a cradle*, and *stand within a masking tape barrier*.

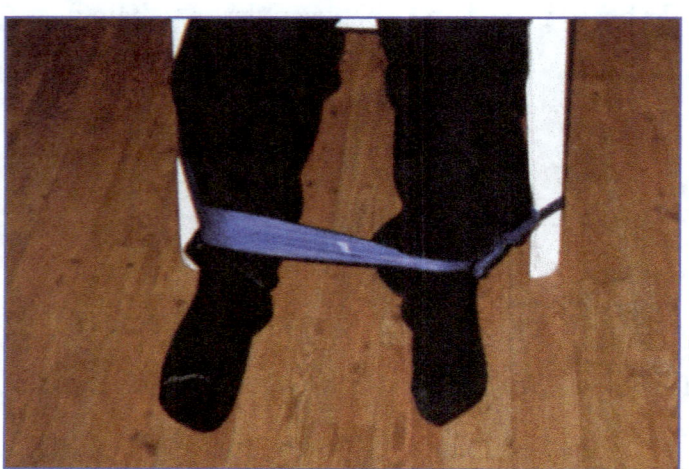

Research supports individual use of the **sit disk** and *therapy ball within a cradle*[15] to increase attention while seated in school.

However, it is also helpful to encourage the student to remain seated without adaptations during less demanding assignments and reward them for paying attention while seated in a regular chair for progressively longer periods. While using these adaptations, therapists or teachers must consider that the students are being prepared to meet the chair-sitting requirements of the teacher they will have the next year. The sit disk and all other listed sitting adaptations make it harder for students to maintain their balance and so should be used only with students who have good balance and who are not gravitationally insecure.

Visual Strategies

Visual supports are often significantly more effective than verbal instructions for students with autism spectrum, developmental, and auditory processing disorders. The third line of environmental

ENVIRONMENTAL ADAPTATION STRATEGIES

adaptations contains visuals. A **visual list** or **visual schedule** provides a foundation that promotes organization and behavior. Each item on the list is put away and checked off before the next is begun. Visual choices and rewards significantly improve students' organizational skills and behavior.[16]

The **visual list** strategy is an effective clinical intervention for teachers and therapists to help organize dysregulated youth who move rapidly from one class or therapy room activity to the next, making a mess and becoming more dysregulated and angry. This technique is also important when teaching students how to follow directions. The therapist or teacher keeps all materials locked up and assists the student in making a sequential list of up to six activities. Students are then given access to the first activity, and they must stay with it for a predetermined minimal amount of time, clean up, and check it off the list before beginning the next task. This cycle repeats for all items on the list. It is sometimes helpful to have the child choose the first activity, the teacher or therapist the second, the child the third, the teacher or therapist the fourth, and so on.

A **visual schedule** uses pictures that help children with developmental disabilities conform to social expectations. Pictures of therapeutic or class activities can help adapt the visual list strategy to the child's developmental level. Picture lists and schedules can be individualized to help students understand tasks, options, routines, rules, transitions, and reinforcement contingencies. Picture schedules can be reviewed before high-risk situations (such as lunchtime or assemblies where the child has previously been physically aggressive) as part of a comprehensive pre-correction strategy.

The **visual if-then** consistently uses picture choices to help students understand what they need to do to earn a preferred activity or a pre-specified reinforcer. The following is an example of if-then for a preferred activity: "If I take off my shoes, then I can play on the swing." A visual if-then for earning a pre-specified reinforcer could be, "If I keep safe hands until lunch, then I earn an extra occupational therapy session after lunch."

A **schedule story** helps children understand and follow new routines and is particularly useful for promoting self-control during transitions in students with developmental challenges. For example, I worked with a first-grade girl who had autism spectrum disorder. She was scheduled to leave the classroom every Monday morning to attend speech and occupational therapy (OT) sessions. The process of leaving the class upset her; she cried and refused to go with the therapists, disrupting the class. With guidance, she developed a schedule story, sequentially describing and drawing pictures of her new routine of leaving her class, attending speech followed by OT, then returning to class. After she constructed the schedule story the therapist repeatedly read it with her, enabling her to follow this new routine.

A second example is a schedule story constructed by a small group of students who were having difficulty choosing and beginning to play their favorite free-time activities. Group members were asked to construct a book, with each student drawing and dictating captions for their favorite free-time activity (e.g., build model airplanes, reading the Barney story). When it was free time the student who liked building models would get the book and select his page. The teacher also copied the build model airplanes page and posted it in the cabinet where the materials to build model airplanes were kept. This process assisted students in independently selecting their favorite free-time activity.

Some classrooms experience many behavior problems. In these cases, finding strategies to increase classroom structure can be immensely helpful in improving self-control in students with complex behavioral challenges. A useful way to recognize the early need for support and to promote direction-following in students with behavioral and attention challenges is the **sit near teacher strategy**. Seating a student close to the teacher's desk enables the student to see the teacher's face and receive close support when directions are given. This technique also encourages the teacher to closely monitor the student.

The **calm face** can help students with hyper-reactivity and low tolerance of frustration increase their self-control. Many students who have complex behavioral challenges show hyper-reactivity of the amygdala.[12] Because the amygdala has extensive connections in responding to facial recognition, tantrums will be worsened if teachers and therapists respond with anger or fear. Therapists and teachers must practice maintaining a calm face when students have tantrums, and they should plan procedures that immediately remove the student from the class or direct the other students to leave the room, because angry or frightened facial reactions among peers can worsen tantrums and reinforce inappropriate behavior.

A particularly helpful strategy for students who have auditory processing difficulties and sensory hyper-reactivity is using **slow speech** and a **slow pace** of teaching. Reducing the pace of instruction provides students with more time to process verbal instructions. These strategies can also reduce anxiety and agitation in students with hyper-reactivity. This may result in less information being presented, but teachers can often reduce their repetition of information or use homework for needed repetition.

However, many students with complex behavioral challenges also have a limited attention span. Instruction needs to be balanced so it is presented slowly enough for them to process while being fast enough to maintain their attention. When working with mainstreamed students, it is also important to not bore students who are rapid auditory processors by overly slowing the auditory pace. An option for classrooms with a limited number of students with auditory processing challenges is to provide these students with simultaneously matching visual information, which allows them to simultaneously hear and read instructions.

The **choice of 1 activity from . . . 4 choices; do ____ minutes minimum; clean up before next activity strategy** can improve self-control while expanding choice-making and attention as foundations for learning. Some students move quickly from one activity to the next, making a mess of the class or therapy room while becoming increasingly dysregulated. The **choice of 1 activity . . . do ____ minutes minimum . . . clean up . . . strategy** addresses individually expanding students' ability to

ENVIRONMENTAL ADAPTATION STRATEGIES

make developmental choices and their attention span while promoting self-control, which can be achieved by structuring them to remain focused on a single activity for a minimal amount of time before proceeding to the next task.

Environmental adaptations provide the structure for improved behavior. Predictable rules and procedures set a safe, reliable structure that enhances self-control. All behavioral improvement efforts begin by reviewing environmental adaptations and modifying them as needed.

CHAPTER 2

SENSORY MODULATION STRATEGIES

Using Sensory Strategies to Improve Behavior

Sensory modulation strategies build on the foundation of environmental adaptation strategies by helping students manage their feelings, arousal levels, and triggers through the use of effective sensory coping strategies. Because most students enjoy sensory activities and like to earn "stuff," they are motivated to use environmental adaptations and sensory modulation strategies. However, it is crucial to integrate sensory modulation with behavioral strategies in order to most effectively improve behavior in students who have complex behavioral challenges.[1]

Sensory modulation strategies for improving behavior can include movement, mindfulness, yoga, and deep-pressure touch interventions. Sensory and behavioral strategies can be integrated to improve behavior in individuals, small groups, and entire classrooms. When using sensory and behavioral strategies in school, therapists and teachers must integrate individual, group, and classroom practices so students with complex behavioral challenges are given a consistent approach that has been proven to improve behavior in school.[2]

Because sensory modulation strategies often confuse teachers, parents, and therapists, I want to clarify the terms and concepts. "Sensory processing" or "sensory integration disorders" are synonymous terms for difficulties organizing, integrating, and functionally using sensory input. Two subcategories of sensory processing disorders most negatively affect behavior: sensory modulation disorder and sensory discrimination disorder. A student with a sensory processing disorder can have a sensory modulation disorder, a sensory discrimination disorder, or both of these challenges.

Sensory modulation disorder makes it difficult to respond to functionally relevant sensory information while ignoring irrelevant input. Sensory modulation strategies help students recognize and adjust their arousal level, thereby improving behavior and learning. A useful assessment for understanding a student's sensory modulation style is the Sensory Profile.

Sensory modulation disorder can include four subcategories of dysfunction:

1. **Sensory over-responsivity** (also referred to as sensory sensitivity and sensory hyper-reactivity) is a significantly high responsiveness to sensory input with neurological difficulty becoming used to sensory input (i.e., habituating). Students who have sensory over-responsivity can use sensory coping strategies to accommodate for the extreme salience of sensory input they experience.[3]

2. **Sensory under-responsivity** (also referred to as sensory hypo-responsivity and low registration) refers to significantly low responsiveness to sensory input, with a tendency to get used to sensory input quickly.

3. **Sensory seeking** is a significant tendency to actively seek out sensory input to the extent that it interferes with learning. It can occur with sensory under-responsivity, as an attempt to self-regulate, but it can also be an ineffective attempt to manage over-responsivity.

4. **Sensory avoidance** is a significant tendency to actively avoid sensory input to the extent that it interferes with learning.

Students with sensory modulation disorder may have one, two, three, or all four of these subcategories of dysfunction. For example, many students with complex behavioral disorders have both significantly high sensory over-responsivity and sensory under-responsivity. These students tend not to notice sensory input, but once they do register a stimulus, they over-respond to it. These students frequently fluctuate between being too under sensitive and too oversensitive to sensory stimuli to behave appropriately. The goal is to assist these students in noticing and adjusting their reactions to maintain an optimal quiet, alert state.

Therapists can incorrectly assume that sensory seeking occurs because a student is experiencing low registration and is not receiving adequate input. While this is true for some students, some sensory-sensitive students engage in sensory-seeking behavior that worsens their hyper-reactivity. If this is the problem for an individual, it is important to structure the environment and teach the student to attend to one activity for as long as possible before switching to another task. The **choice of 1 activity from ____ choices; do ____ minutes minimum . . . clean up . . . strategy** described in Chapter 1 is particularly useful for these students. This strategy helps them remain focused on a single activity rather than engaging in sensory-seeking behavior that worsens their sensory sensitivity.

While behavioral disorders are different from sensory modulation disorders, students with developmental and behavioral disorders are significantly more likely to also have sensory modulation

SENSORY MODULATION STRATEGIES

disorders. If students have both behavioral and sensory modulation disorders, the two difficulties need to be addressed simultaneously for improved learning. Research indicates that only 5 percent of typical students have sensory modulation disorders, whereas more than 50 percent of students with autism spectrum disorders and one-third with post-traumatic stress disorder[4] or mental illness have sensory modulation disorders. Because so many students with complex behavioral disorders have sensory modulation challenges, it is important to assess whether students with complex behavioral disorders *do* experience these challenges, and if so, to address them.

Sensory over-responsivity challenges are most important to address in students with complex behavioral challenges. Research indicates that students with sensory over-responsivity (where only 2 percent of children the same age score) are significantly more likely to have behavioral problems than children who do not have sensory over-responsivity.[5] Recent research specifically found that students with autism spectrum disorders and anxiety disorder as well as sensory over-responsivity have significantly low neurological habituation (e.g., the amygdala and primary sensory cortices are not fully able to regulate auditory and tactile inputs).[6]

Tactile defensiveness refers to an over-responsivity to touch. This can cause students to perceive light touch as painful. In addition, when they are physically close to others, they may feel uncomfortable because they are more likely to be unexpectedly touched, and this can contribute to behavioral problems. For example, a student might punch a child who brushes up against them because the light touch is irritating or painful. Tactile defensiveness can also interfere with early childhood learning activities; for example, students may resist getting haircuts or playing tag because they dislike being touched.

Gravitational insecurity refers to an over-responsivity to movement. In extreme forms this can make students fearful of using swings or even of walking. Research supports a relation between gravitational insecurity and fearful, neurotic behavior.[7]

Sensory discrimination disorder is the second main category of sensory processing disorder that also seems to negatively affect behavior. Sensory discrimination disorder involves difficulties identifying, differentiating, interpreting, and organizing input from the various senses. Sensory discrimination disorder negatively affects body awareness and organizational skills. Body awareness difficulties are more common in students with post-traumatic stress disorder (PTSD) and autism spectrum disorders. Students with poor body awareness or organizational difficulties find it harder to develop self-esteem, personal boundaries, self-control, and social skills, as well as to plan movements.

Sensory discrimination disorder can involve any of the sensory systems: tactile (touch), proprioceptive (muscle force/tension), interoceptive (internal states such as hunger, soreness), olfactory (smell), gustatory (taste), auditory, and visual. The most widely known sensory discrimination problem is tactile discrimination disorder, in which students lack body awareness through touch.

Students with sensory discrimination disorder often have body image difficulties, move awkwardly, appear to have low muscle tone, lean on walls and other people, and are reluctant to interact in unfamiliar activities. A third-grader with sensory discrimination disorder created this illustration; she was asked to cut out and assemble random body parts to form a picture of a girl. This student was bright but demonstrated an inability to identify which of her fingers I was touching without using her vision. Her art project shows a disorganized body scheme, with asymmetrical orientation of the eyes and ears.

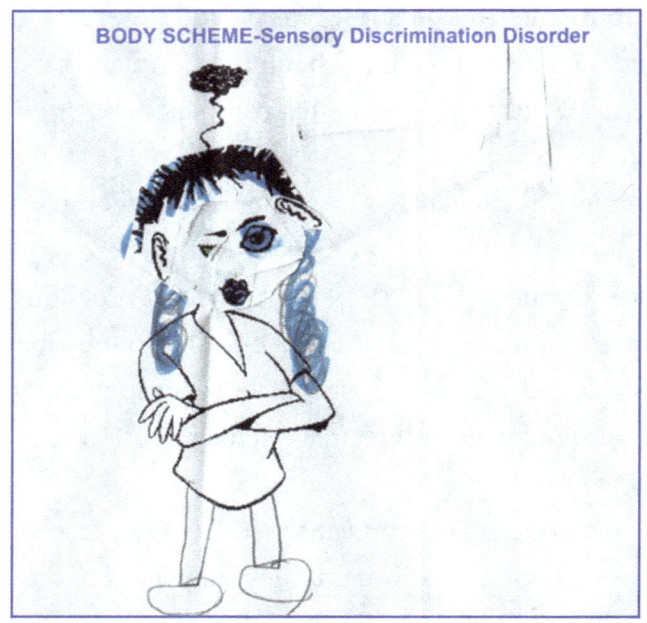

Sensory discrimination disorder involves difficulty organizing and integrating input from the various senses. For example, a student may become disorganized and confused when attempting to write on a whiteboard the answer to a teacher's verbal question. Difficulties may result when the students tries to functionally organize and integrate the auditory input of the question with the proprioceptive and visual senses involved in the movement and vision required for writing the answer, along with the squeaking sound and smell of the marker.[8]

Assessments Guiding Sensory Strategies

A useful clinical tool for determining the function of problematic behaviors is the Questions About Behavior Function (QABF) form. If the QABF form indicates that students are exhibiting problem behavior to obtain attention; to escape tasks, work, or physical discomfort; or both, functional communication training (FCT) can be used to determine a more appropriate behavior for expressing these needs. These needs can be expressed through the use of verbal or sign language mands and other individualized communication strategies.

Alternatively, if students are doing inappropriate repetitive behaviors primarily for the sensory input they provide, it is best to find an alternative, more appropriate way for them to obtain this input. For example, if a student is rocking back and forth in his seat because he enjoys the movement sensation and the rocking distracts others in the class, the student can be given a rocking chair to sit in while doing classwork. If possible, it is best for mental health, behavioral, occupational, and speech/language therapists to collaborate with the teacher in finding the most useful strategies.

SENSORY MODULATION STRATEGIES

Brief practical assessments that can be used to guide selection of the most appropriate FAB Strategies include the Sensory Profile, finger identification test, FAB Trigger & Coping forms, preference assessment, and Questions About Behavioral Function (QABF). The information obtained with these forms should be integrated with the student's medical, academic achievement, and developmental assessments.

Because students with developmental, mental health, and behavioral challenges are significantly likely to have sensory modulation difficulties, it is important to assess and provide, if needed, intervention to address them.[9] The Sensory Profile is a reliable, valid assessment that identifies significantly different sensory modulation. Sensory Profile scores showing a definite difference from those of others (e.g., a considerable difference from age-matched peers is found for only two of one hundred students) indicate that a student has a particular sensory modulation characteristic. Versions of the Sensory Profile are available for individuals from infancy through adulthood, and the newest version distinguishes between sensory and behavioral challenges.[10]

Sensory modulation strategies are important for students with behavioral challenges because the students are often motivated to do the activities. Once a client learns to recognize when they are in a dysfunctional high-arousal state, therapists can coach them on applying appropriate emotion-regulation strategies that are based on their interests, developmental level, and goals. Significant sensory modulation difficulties in auditory filtering, low registration/sensory seeking, and tactile sensitivity were related to attention and academic achievement challenges. These students benefited from developing coping strategies to improve their attention, learning, and behavior. It is helpful to combine the Sensory Profile, Trigger and Coping forms, behavioral function assessments, and behavioral preference assessments when determining the best teaching and reinforcement strategies.[11]

The finger identification test is a tactile discrimination assessment item from the Miller Assessment for Preschoolers that is useful for identifying extreme sensory discrimination disorder. This item asks students to identify which finger is touched while keeping their eyes closed. Assessment norms indicate that children should be able to consistently and accurately identify which finger is touched by three years old. Some high school students with PTSD who are academically above grade level fail this assessment item. Interventions for sensory discrimination disorder are most effective after a quiet alert state has been achieved.

The FAB Trigger & Coping forms is both an assessment and intervention tool. Use of the FAB Trigger & Coping forms and similar safety tools empower students to recognize triggers of their inappropriate behavior and to instead use their most effective coping strategy. Use of the FAB Trigger & Coping forms and the recommended coping strategies can significantly reduce student arousal levels and the incidence of both seclusion and restraint.[12] The FAB Trigger & Coping forms is described and can be downloaded for use at fabstrategies.org/2018/12/07/fab-trigger-coping-forms. The FAB

FAB FUNCTIONALLY ALERT BEHAVIOR STRATEGIES

Trigger & Coping forms can be included as a component of occupational, physical, speech/language, or mental health therapy assessments and enables therapists to promote motivation by introducing students to new coping strategies while assessing their awareness of their triggers and coping strategies. The pictures from the FAB Trigger & Coping strategies form can also be used to construct coping cards and other visual supports displaying the student's coping strategies. A student preference assessment enables therapists and teachers to identify what activities students like and are motivated to do. Simple preference assessments involve simultaneously offering a student two toys or activities and noting which one they select.

The Questions About Behavioral Function (QABF) assessment is a useful tool that helps therapists and teachers make sure that their sensory interventions will improve, rather than worsen, a student's specific aggressive or inappropriate behavior. Students misbehave for a reason. It is important to understand the need that a student's inappropriate behavior is meeting in order to determine the most effective interventions for promoting appropriate behavior.[13]

Sensory modulation strategies were developed to improve students' functioning, but research found that sensory strategies increase the behaviors they directly follow.[14] Because sensory strategies are reinforcing they can unintentionally increase inappropriate behaviors. An understanding of why students are engaging in inappropriate behavior is necessary to ensure that sensory strategies do not unintentionally reinforce and worsen problematic behavior.[15]

The QABF assessment is a quick and easy tool for guiding therapists and teachers in their use of sensory strategies. The QABF helps identify whether the primary function of a behavior is to escape demands or discomfort, obtain attention, obtain objects, or get sensory stimulation. As will be further discussed in Chapter 6, it is crucial for occupational therapists to obtain a functional behavioral analysis assessment to assure that sensory intervention does not accidentally reinforce inappropriate behavior. Because his QABF assessment (shown on the next page) indicates that the self-injurious behavior is primarily being done for nonsocial, automatic sensory reinforcement, it suggests that use of a sensory replacement behavior will be helpful.

Case study research suggests that combining behavior function, sensory modulation, and preference assessments can guide the use of sensory strategies to significantly improve behavior in students with severe behavioral challenges.[11] Unfortunately, this combination of assessments through collaboration between therapists and teachers is insufficiently implemented.

Once a student's Sensory Profile, developmental, and needs assessment is completed, it is helpful to consider the student's individual environmental triggers, body triggers, and coping strategies related to their problematic behavior. Therapists are helpful during this process because they can simultaneously conduct a developmental and a preference assessment to ensure that learning tasks both interest the student and are at the appropriate developmental level, rather than only the correct academic or chronological age level. Students often have developmental, sensory modulation, sensory

SENSORY MODULATION STRATEGIES

Student's Name: *13 yr. old c̄ ASD, ODD & Attachment Disorder;*
Definite Difference SP = Low Reg & Sensory Seeking
Date: _____

Behavior: *Head banging against the floor*   Respondent: *John Pagano, PhD, OTR/L*

QUESTIONS ABOUT BEHAVIORAL FUNCTION (QABF)

Rate how often the student demonstrates the behaviors in situations where they might occur. Be sure to rate how often each behavior occurs, not what you think a good answer would be.

X = Doesn't apply   0 = Never   1 = Rarely   2 – Some   3 = Often

Score	Number	Behavior
0	1.	Engages in the behavior to get attention.
0	2.	Engages in the behavior to escape work or learning situations.
3	3.	Engages in the behavior as a form of "self-stimulation".
1	4.	Engages in the behavior because he/she is in pain.
0	5.	Engages in the behavior to get access to items such as preferred toys, food, or beverages.
0	6.	Engages in the behavior because he/she likes to be reprimanded.
0	7.	Engages in the behavior when asked to do something (get dressed, brush teeth, work, etc.)
3	8.	Engages in the behavior even if he/she thinks no one is in the room.
2	9.	Engages in the behavior more frequently when he/she is ill.
0	10.	Engages in the behavior when you take something away from him/her.
0	11.	Engages in the behavior to draw attention to himself/herself.
0	12.	Engages in the behavior when he/she does not want to do something.
2	13.	Engages in the behavior because there is nothing else to do.
1	14.	Engages in the behavior when there is something bothering him/her physically.
0	15.	Engages in the behavior when you have something that he/she wants.
0	16.	Engages in the behavior to try to get a reaction from you.
0	17.	Engages in the behavior to try to get people to leave him/her alone.
3	18.	Engages in the behavior in a highly repetitive manner, ignoring his/her surroundings.
1	19.	Engages in the behavior because he/she is physically uncomfortable.
0	20.	Engages in the behavior when a peer has something that he/she wants.
0	21.	Does he/she seem to be saying, "come see me" or "look at me" when engaging in the behavior?
0	22.	Does he/she seem to be saying, "leave me alone" or "stop asking me to do this" when engaging in the behavior?
3	23.	Does he/she seem to enjoy the behavior, even if no one is around?
1	24.	Does the behavior seem to indicate to you that he/she is not feeling well?
0	25.	Does he/she seem to be saying, "give me that (toy, food, item)" when engaging in the behavior?

Attention	Escape	Non-social *Sensory*	Physical	Tangible
1. Attention: 0	2. Escape: 0	3. Self-stim: 3	4. In pain: 1	5. Access to items: 0
6. Reprimand: 0	7. Do something: 0	8. Thinks alone: 3	9. When ill: 2	10. Takes away: 0
11. Draws: 0	12. Not do: 0	13. Nothing to do: 2	14. Physical problem: 1	15. You have: 0
16. Reaction: 0	17. Alone: 0	18. Repetitive: 3	19. Uncomfortable: 1	20. Peer has: 0
21. "Come see": 0	22. "Leave alone": 0	23. Enjoy by self: 2	24. Not feeling well: 1	25. "Give me that": 0
Total: 0	Total: 0	Total: 13	Total: 6	Total: 0

Sensory - Automatic

Revised 4-19-01

(Reprinted with permission from Johnny Matson, Ph.D.)

discrimination, mental health, PTSD, and early attachment challenges that affect their behavioral problems. Developmental assessment is important because it assesses their cognitive, receptive language, expressive language, and social skills, along with specific trials with communication supports. The first step is defining problematic behavior and having the student and family consider what environmental and body triggers precede the behavior, as well as what effective coping strategies the student is already using.

It is empowering to involve students, their families, and therapists/teachers in assessing environmental triggers, body triggers, and the most effective coping strategies for avoiding problematic behaviors. The student, staff, and family are empowered by reviewing what they already know precedes and reduces the problematic behavior. Trigger and coping strategies with visual supports can guide students in recognizing and managing their arousal level and emotions for improved short- and long-term functioning.

Intervention Using Sensory Modulation Strategies

The term "sensory-based interventions" (SBIs) is commonly used to describe environmental adaptation, sensory modulation, and physical self-regulation strategies listed on the FAB Strategies form. SBIs are specific, goal-directed adaptive equipment and sensory strategies that improve behavior by addressing sensory modulation and sensory discrimination challenges. SBIs can be useful for preventing incidents of inappropriate behavior or teaching replacement activities that decrease aggressive and self-injurious behavior.

SBIs are widely used in early intervention programs, schools, group homes, psychiatric hospitals, and juvenile justice settings. They can be provided through individual, group, and consultative interventions. While randomly or consistently applying SBIs to all clients with behavioral challenges is described as "sensory-based intervention," in this book the term is limited to the use of specific, goal-directed behavioral improvement that is based on individualized assessment.

SBIs help occupational, speech/language, physical, and mental health therapists to guide parents and teachers in embedding goal-directed strategies into the student's daily routine. It is best to repeatedly embed SBIs into the daily routine to avoid aggression and to reinforce students for applying them. The FAB Strategies form was developed to provide an efficient way for therapists to coordinate with other teachers and professionals on the consistent use of individualized SBIs to help students. SBIs have been integrated into many developmental, educational, and behavior support interventions.

SBIs are a major component of the evidence-based Sensory Motor Arousal Regulation Treatment (SMART) and Attachment, Regulation and Competency (ARC) framework for youth with PTSD,

SENSORY MODULATION STRATEGIES

the Floortime Approach for improving behavior of students with autism spectrum disorder, the Collaborative Problem Solving Approach for oppositional defiant disorder, the Alert Program for improving self-regulation in youth with fetal alcohol syndrome, and the Zones of Regulation program for students with self-regulation challenges.

SBIs offer occupational therapy practitioners a tool for expanding their role in schools by providing more group and consultative interventions in naturalistic school environments. Many FAB Strategies are SBIs, especially those in the environmental adaptation and sensory modulation sections of the form. Occupational therapy practitioners can integrate SBIs with the psychosocial, developmental, and occupational frames of reference in applying evidence-based interventions that are embedded in classroom and school learning activities. School occupational therapy practitioners can also integrate visual supports with SBI strategies to guide students, school personnel, and parents in regulating arousal levels for improved learning.

It is important to clearly distinguish SBIs from sensory integration therapy (SIT). Also referred to as Ayres Sensory Integration, SIT uses clinic-based, child-directed activities that adhere to designated core concepts involving sensory interactions to facilitate an adaptive response. While both SBIs and SIT are based on sensory integration theory, they are different interventions that have distinct research support. Clinic referrals for SIT can be extremely helpful when youth are initially discharged from mental health hospitals or group homes to home settings. Note, however, that SIT interventions are not listed on the FAB Strategies form.

If students with complex behavioral challenges have both sensory modulation and sensory discrimination disorders, it is important for therapists and teachers to first assist them in becoming aware of their sensory modulation difficulties and helping them achieve a quiet, alert state. In a student with sensory modulation and complex behavioral challenges, sensory modulation strategies can significantly improve self-regulation and reduce distress by teaching the student to monitor and use coping strategies to adjust their arousal level. Students who have sensory modulation disorder can be taught to notice whether their arousal level is too high (hyper and fidgety) or too low (sleepy and sluggish) to learn and behave in school, and then to use coping strategies to adjust their level appropriately. Most students learn best when in a quiet, alert state, rather than when they are overly excited or drowsy.

Maintaining an appropriate arousal level is also a social skill, because arousal level expectations are different depending on the environment (e.g., higher arousal level expectations exist in physical education than in reading classes). The main difference I've found between students with sensory modulation disorder who are successful and those who are in juvenile detention facilities is their ability to adjust their arousal level to the environment. Students must practice often in order to be able to independently adjust their arousal level to a constantly changing environment.

Before beginning an intervention, it is also extremely important to assess the degree to which a student prefers specific environmental adaptation and sensory modulation strategies and how they can be used in teaching, in treatment, and as reinforcement. It is also important to understand how a specific environmental adaptation or sensory modulation strategy relates to the function of problematic behavior.

Sensory Modulation Strategies on the FAB Strategies Form

Many of the sensory modulation strategies listed in Section B of the FAB Strategies form simultaneously address sensory modulation and sensory discrimination challenges. These strategies are from diverse frames of reference, including SBI, physical exercise, movement, progressive relaxation, stretching, mindfulness, yoga, and massage. The sensory modulation strategies involving massage, referred to as FAB Pressure Touch Strategies, are described in Chapter 3.

The arousal level and arousal level modify strategies are a unique integration of the ARC trauma energy levels, Zones of Regulation,[16] and traffic light behavior systems commonly used in schools. The **modulate arousal level** strategy can be done during both individual and group interventions to help students become aware of their current arousal level and recognize whether it is functional for their current tasks. In the traffic light system, arousal level is taught using three traffic lights that are consistent with the colors and descriptions of other arousal level systems but are easier to learn. These traffic lights are integrated with sensory modulation arousal levels and smells to make them easy to learn with a multisensory approach.

The **modulate arousal level strategy** teaches students individualized coping strategies to manage their arousal level for improved behavior. Research indicates that students with sensory modulation and behavioral disorders can benefit from environmental adaptations and individualized sensory coping strategies to manage their neurologically based lack of habituation to sensory input. Research supports the efficacy of teaching students to identify and use sensory coping strategies that are embedded in their daily routines in order to manage their arousal level for improved behavior and learning.[17]

Students with behavioral and sensory modulation challenges need sensory activities to replace their current dysfunctional "coping" strategies for managing uncomfortable energy levels (e.g., cutting themselves, banging their head). Motor learning research suggests that it is easiest to stop dysfunctional behaviors by repeatedly replacing them with new, highly preferred activities that are embedded in daily routines (e.g., rubbing arms with a scrub brush to replace cutting, massaging the head to replace banging it). These new strategies help clients manage their sensory modulation and behavioral challenges.

In contrast, if a student has little energy and is too lethargic to learn, he can do jumping jacks or take a walk to increase his alertness for improved learning. In this way, coping strategies are

SENSORY MODULATION STRATEGIES

Arousal Level

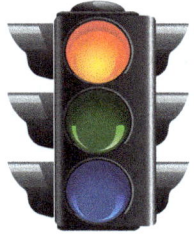 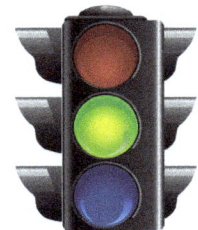 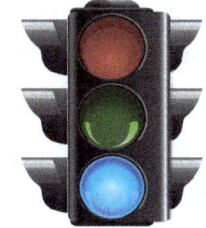

Over-Responsive

Cherry Scent

Quiet Alert Responsive

Apple Scent

Under-Responsive

Blueberry Scent

Copyright © 2019 by John Pagano, Ph.D., OTR/L, www.fabstrategies.org
Permission granted for direct use with clients.

implemented so children learn, with adult assistance, to modulate their energy level up and down as needed. Energy modulation is an advanced strategy that takes several months of regular practice to learn. For the first couple of months, the student is repeatedly directed to notice and rate their energy level. The students' therapists and teachers can best teach the concepts of energy level and energy level modulation by first assisting the student in recognizing when their energy level begins to slightly increase and then modulating it (e.g., by doing push-ups).

When students describe their arousal level as "hyper-responsive and comfortable" or appear resistant to a therapist's or teacher's efforts to reduce their energy level, the students usually are uncomfortable in a quiet alert state, either because they're unaccustomed to being in a quiet, alert state or previously experienced trauma when they were in such a state (e.g., at night when relaxed for bed). In these cases the therapist is more likely to be successful in reducing the student's energy level if they proceed gradually. It can also be helpful to initially practice a new coping strategy in an extremely safe environment such as the sensory coping area or during individual therapy.[18]

Event triggers, *body triggers*, and **coping strategies** are the main sensory strategies used in conjunction with energy level modulation strategies to help clients learn to use coping strategies to replace inappropriate behavior. *Event triggers* are specific environmental situations that precede inappropriate behavior, such as being told "no." To visually learn emotional regulation strategies, students can draw and post pictures to distinguish appropriate feelings from inappropriate behaviors. This enables students to identify and build on their existing awareness of triggers and effective coping strategies.

Body triggers are the physical cues such as sweating, hand fisting, and acting mean or rude. Teachers and therapists can help students become aware of these as signals preceding inappropriate behavior. Repeatedly educating students and their teachers about individual environmental and body triggers helps students to avoid the antecedents of inappropriate behaviors or anticipate their need for coping strategies.

Coping strategies are individualized, preferred sensory activities that address sensory modulation challenges, modulate arousal, and replace inappropriate behavior. It is easiest to stop dysfunctional habits by repeatedly replacing them with more functional activities that are embedded in the daily routine. It is useful to begin with coping strategies that students are already using (as identified on the FAB Trigger & Coping form). If additional coping strategies are needed to manage "big feelings," it is helpful to use body-oriented movement strategies, such as "feeling your feet" or doing push-ups.[19]

It is important to teach and reinforce students for using coping strategies on a daily basis and to manage crisis situations, as seemingly harmless sensory events associated with a past trauma frequently trigger students with PTSD.[20] Routine use of favorite coping strategies, such as taking a walk, can be integrated into these students' daily routine to reduce both arousal and incidents of inappropriate behavior. Students can use strategies for coping with crisis, such as doing push-ups in the sensory coping area, to prevent inappropriate behavior when they experience environmental and body triggers. Teaching students with PTSD and sensory modulation difficulties to use routine and crisis sensory coping strategies to modulate their arousal level significantly improved their behavior.[21]

Mindfulness FAB Strategies

A variety of mindfulness FAB Strategies are described in this section; these are useful for reducing stress and improving self-control and attention in students with PTSD and other mental health challenges.[22] These strategies are presented in developmental sequence from easiest to most difficult so that each can be individualized to each student's developmental level. It is important to match the strategy with the student's or class's preferences and developmental abilities. The goal is for students to learn mindfulness strategies they enjoy and that are easy enough for them to do but also are difficult enough that they have to give their full attention to the activity and can't think of anything else.

The **hand breathing** strategy is taught in a developmentally progressive sequence that is especially useful for students at a preschool and kindergarten developmental level and students who have

SENSORY MODULATION STRATEGIES

difficulty with hand cramping while writing. **Hand breathing** begins by having students imitate the therapist in slowly opening their hands while stretching and separating their fingers, then gradually closing their hands to make a fist. Hand breathing progresses to include breathing in as the hands are opened, so the hands are fully opened and the fingers separated when the student has completely inhaled, then gradually breathing out so their hands are in fists (with the thumb inside) upon full exhalation. Finally, this

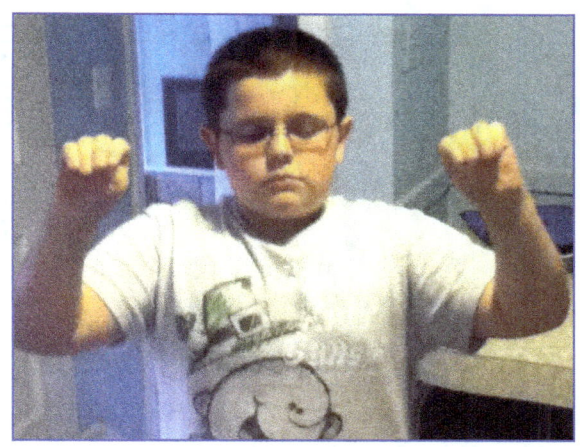

strategy is made most challenging by having students make the exhalation longer than the inhalation. In mindfulness practice, breathing out slower than in increases relaxation. Hand breathing includes Adi Mudra, wherein the thumb is placed on the palm under the pinky and the other fingers are closed over it, forming a fist; this can be specifically helpful for encouraging calmness.

Bird breathing is a simple mindfulness activity that is first taught by having students vertically raise then lower their arms. Next, breathing is added: Students inhale as they gradually raise their arms and exhale as they gradually lower their arms. Then the exhalation is made slower and longer than the inhalation. If the students chose to make bird sounds, they must be made silently, so the class is not disturbed.

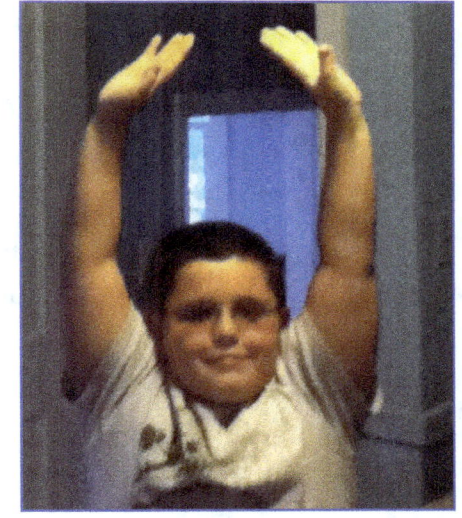

Stretch down begins with students standing with both feet aligned shoulder-width apart and the knees straight. Then they lower their hands toward the floor. From the bent position, students interlace their fingers and vertically *stretch up* toward the sky as their feet press downward into the ground. From the *stretch up* position, they move to the left side, then the right, for ten seconds for *stretch lateral*. From *stretch up*, they twist their entire body to each side as far as possible and hold for ten seconds in *stretch rotation*.

Neck circles involve clients making circular motions with their neck, three rotations in each direction. *Shoulder circles* involve clients making circular motions with their shoulder blades: up, back, then down for three rotations. *Hip circles* involve clients making circular motions with their hips, three rotations in each direction, then doing a figure-eight movement with their hips, three times in each direction. These types of basic exercises, as well as the progressive relaxation and mindfulness strategies described in the next section, are often helpful initial considerations for highly distressed students who need to learn basic coping strategies.

FAB FUNCTIONALLY ALERT BEHAVIOR STRATEGIES

Progressive Relaxation and Mindfulness Strategies

Tense and relax is a brief progressive relaxation strategy involving the three muscle groups students most often tense when they're anxious:

1. Tense, then relax, all the muscles of your face and jaw.

2. Elevate both shoulders toward your ears, then drop and relax both shoulders.

3. Fist hands tightly, then completely relax both wrists, hands, and fingers.

In each step, participants tense their muscles for three seconds then relax them for five to ten seconds, doing each step three times.

The strategy called **4–4–6–2 breathing** is a breath-counting mindfulness strategy that can be useful for teachers, therapists, and high-functioning students. It can also help students with mental health challenges whose medications are being reduced or changed. This 4–4–6–2 breath-counting strategy begins by having students inhale for a count of four, then exhale for a count of six. Then students are sequentially prompted to hold their breath for four seconds after the inhale, and two seconds after the exhale.

The more advanced form of **4–4–6–2 breathing** requires students to breathe in for a count of four, hold the breath for a count of four, breathe out for a count of four, and hold the exhalation for a count of two. This strategy requires a lot of concentration, but by redirecting a student's attention from the source of anger to counting breaths, it can help the student calm down when they are upset.

Many mindfulness movement strategies can be taught as individual and group interventions, initially taught by therapists when pulling a student out of the classroom, then done with the entire class once the child with special needs is familiar with the activity. The **mindful clock sit strategy** was found to improve self-control in first-grade students, particularly those with behavioral challenges.[23] The specific sequence can be sequentially introduced to help irritable students develop a basic sensory awareness of the front-back, top-bottom, and lateral orientations of their body. It involves verbalizing specific words (designated in **bold** print below) while moving in a specific sequence (described in *italics*) to promote basic awareness of the front, back, top, and bottom of the body. Students complete the entire sequence three times.

Tic *sway forward* **Toc** *sway back* **Like a** *sway forward* **Clock** *sway back*

Till we *sway forward* **Find our** *sway back* **Center** *assume a centered sitting position*

SENSORY MODULATION STRATEGIES

Tic *sway left* **Toc** *sway right* **Like a** *sway left* **Clock** *sway right*

Till we *sway left* **Find our** *sway right* **Center** *assume a centered sitting position*[24]

The **mindful clock stand strategy** is also useful for promoting mindfulness and basic body awareness, and is particularly helpful for students who dislike breathing mindfulness activities. As in the similar sit strategy, the specific sequence can help irritable students who lack sensory awareness of their bodily orientations. The chant verbalizes specific words (designated in **bold** print) while the body moves in a specific sequence (described in *italics*) to promote basic awareness of the front, back, top and bottom of the body. Students complete the entire sequence three times.

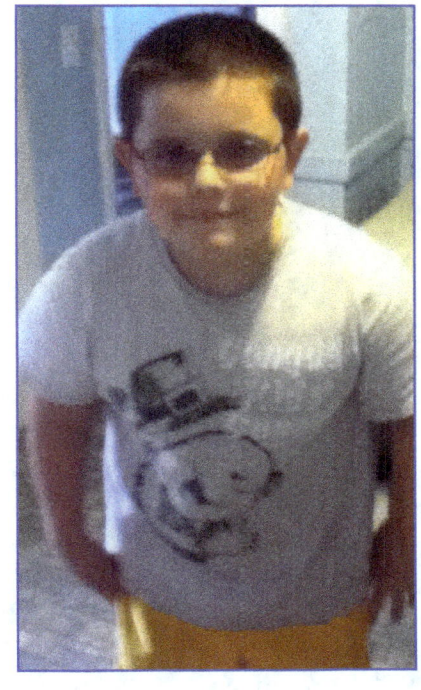

Tic *squat* **Toc** *stand on toes* **Like a** *squat* **Clock** *stand on toes*

Till we *squat* **Find our** *stand on toes* **Center** *assume a centered standing position*

Tic *lean forward* **Toc** *lean back* **Like a** *lean forward* **Clock** *lean back*

Till we *lean forward* **Find our** *lean back* **Center** *assume a centered standing position*

Focus on feet and *focus on palms* are two body-oriented mindfulness strategies that can be useful in improving body image, decreasing aggression, managing anxiety, and controlling obsessive thoughts. They are mindfulness activities that enable students to calm themselves by redirecting their attention from what is angering them to their body. Research supports that the *focus on feet* strategy significantly reduces physical and verbal aggression in students with conduct disorder,[25] mild intellectual disability,[26] and autism spectrum disorder.[27]

The *focus on feet* strategy trains students to systematically focus all their attention on the bottom of their feet, and it can initially be combined with simultaneously pressing down on or vibrating their feet. Students are asked to close their eyes and feel one foot by concentrating their attention on their big toe, the smaller toe next to it, the center toe, the second smallest toe, and finally the little toe. Students "feel" their toes, bend them, and notice whether they have socks on and whether there are holes in their socks. Next they can move their attention to the ball of their foot, then farther back to feel their arch and notice whether it hits the ground, then to feel their heel.

FAB FUNCTIONALLY ALERT BEHAVIOR STRATEGIES

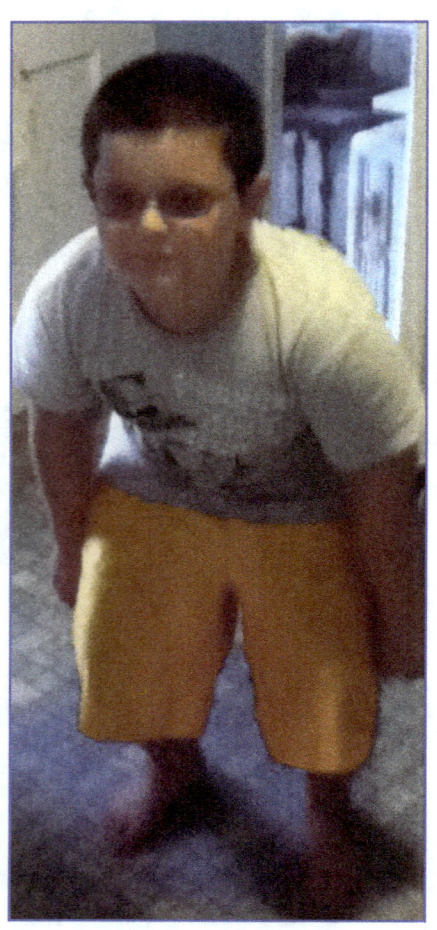

Finally, students are asked to feel or press down on the entire bottom of their foot.

The *focus on palms* strategy teaches students mindfulness through body awareness. Students put their open hands together in prayer position then push them together forcefully for ten seconds, doing an isometric contraction. After this, both hands are held palms up while the eyes are closed. Students sequentially concentrate on feeling their thumb, pointer, middle, ring, and little fingers. They then feel the palms of the hands for five to ten seconds.

Focus on palms can be taught directly after both hands are isometrically pressed together; then the therapist can guide the child through concentrating on feeling the palms. Once the child learns focus on feet or palms, they practice the structured use of this method in a graded manner (e.g., initially throughout the day when there is no stress; next in situations of planned slight stress, such as waiting in line or losing at a game; and finally in moderately stressful situations such as being told "no").

The *body scan* builds on the *focus on feet and palms* strategy to concentrate body awareness on all the major body parts on both sides of the body, reducing arousal while improving body awareness. Tell the children that a golden butterfly is landing on various parts of their body while emitting a calming, empowering light. The body scan proceeds with the golden butterfly landing on their head and then flying to land individually onto each shoulder, hand, knee, and foot.

A guided mindfulness strategy that is useful individually or in groups with children experiencing prolonged anger and loneliness is *kindness*. Children are guided to visualize various people and wish them health, safety, and happiness. The method begins by visualizing a person or animal toward whom the child feels unconditional love, next visualizing an acquaintance, and finally themselves. This technique can gradually help clients develop compassion and empathy for themselves and others.

Basic body awareness is the foundation for helping students with sensory discrimination disorder. A developmental approach that is extremely useful for clients who have a history of PTSD, sensory discrimination disorders, autism spectrum disorders, or all three, is to give them basic body awareness through mindfulness, movement, and touch strategies. The first clinical step in developing basic body awareness is the *sensory front-back top-bottom strategy.*

When leading a small group of students who are resistant to lowering their energy level, it is best to start activities at the group's current energy level, then gradually decreasing the intensity of

SENSORY MODULATION STRATEGIES

activities to guide them toward a more optimal quiet, alert state. For example, if a group resisted doing calming mindfulness activities, the therapist could incrementally reduce their energy level by beginning the **mindful clock sit strategy** at a very rapid pace then gradually slowing it to a rapid pace. In this example the goal would be to try to initially transition the students from extremely hyper to only hyper. The most reliable way I have found to lower energy is to ask a student to apply deep pressure through the body's joints using a slow, linear movement, such as doing push-ups or pushing linearly on a swing.

Freeze dance and *freeze shake* involve standing and seated movements, respectively, that need to stop when the music or drumming stops, then restart when they resume, following the beat if possible. **Giant steps** involve participants asking "may I" to get permission before following the stated sequence of movements (e.g., hops, small or giants steps forward or backward). **Simon says** allows movements to be copied only when Simon says and to be inhibited all other times. *Red light* requires movement to stop at a red light, slow down at a yellow light, and resume at a green light. It can involve movement on a trampoline, Jump-O-Lene, or during any therapy task. All these strategies work on inhibitory motor control, an important but overlooked skill, students should develop in order to decrease aggression. Impulsive aggression, which is particularly common among students with sensory over-responsivity and ADHD, is a main factor discriminating between aggressive and nonaggressive adolescents.[28] All of these strategies are a fun way to address a student's inhibitory motor control. The games *hokey pokey* and *Twister* practice inhibitory motor control and sensory discrimination through body awareness and the simultaneous integration of multiple sensory inputs (sound, movement, proprioception, and touch).

Deliver books, **deliver messages**, and **deliver box** (usually filled with books or other heavy items) are three activities that provide deep pressure through the joints to improve behavior;[29] all three can be embedded into the classroom routine. Deliver books, messages, and a box each combine slow, linear movement with deep pressure through the joints based on clinical sensory integration principles, suggesting that this combined proprioceptive and vestibular input improves body awareness, sensory modulation, and organized behavior.

Rolling to read and **rolling to math** are strategies for students with advanced cognitive abilities but who have difficulties with seated attention. In resource room, homework, as well as occupational, physical, and speech/language therapy sessions, their advanced reading and math skills can be practiced by having them roll across the floor or rug and back, then read a book chapter or do ten math flash cards.

These two strategies alternate academic skills with vestibular and deep-pressure input that allows for active movement and behavioral organization. Finally, allowing breaks from academic work to *draw* and do *crafts* can provide breaks between subjects, allowing students to process information, and fun times during which to practice bilateral skills (holding the paper while drawing or making

31

FAB FUNCTIONALLY ALERT BEHAVIOR STRATEGIES

crafts, but allowing the paper to be taped or using a clipboard during writing assignments to minimize frustration).

A *feeling wheel* is a constructed art project that allows for visual depiction of basic feelings. The student colors in the feelings depicted on the feeling wheel, cuts out the wheel and arrow, pastes the wheel on cardboard, laminates it, then uses a brad to attach the arrow. After they make their feeling wheel, a student can be asked to move the arrow to indicate their current feelings. The *feeling wheel* can also be used to teach students to demonstrate and identify feelings. Students spin the arrow then act out the feeling indicated. The first student to identify the feeling being acted out gets to go next. Feelings are best learned by using a developmental sequence, with mad, sad, and glad taught first. Once children understand these feelings, they can be taught others, such as tense, scared, surprised, disgusted, and relaxed.

Feelings vs. behavior involves a visual representation, using drawings or pictures cut out from worksheets or magazines, that lists feelings on one side of the paper (e.g., mad, sad, glad) and inappropriate behaviors (e.g., kick, bite, swear) on the other. It clarifies for students that it is important to be aware of and experience their feelings, which are normal experiences that increase awareness. However, this strategy also clarifies that behaviors are different than feelings, and that some behaviors are unacceptable in certain or all situations.

The final aspect of the FAB energy modulation strategy is embedding into the daily routine individualized strategies that effectively manage students' energy levels, and the automatic practice of recognizing early signs of triggers and automatically engaging in coping strategies. Practice with coping strategies can begin in the sensory coping area, where the environment can be easily managed. Deep-pressure activities with slow, linear movements (e.g., "wheelbarrow" walking on hands over a therapy ball) are frequently helpful for modulating energy levels. Daily cardiovascular (e.g., an hour-long walk, a half-hour jog), relaxation (e.g., thirty minutes of meditation, mindfulness activities, or yoga), and heavy work or other physical activities (lawn mowing, weightlifting, swimming) often help clients maintain a quiet, alert state.

The *decrease, then if needed, gradually increase sensory input strategy* is a simple guideline that can help all students regulate their arousal level to improve behavior and learning, regardless of their specific subcategories of sensory modulation dysfunction. It is important that students with sensory modulation difficulties, autism spectrum disorder, PTSD, or mental illness be given assistance as needed to maintain a quiet, alert state before beginning other behavioral interventions.

If a student has any or all types of sensory modulation disorder (e.g., under-responsivity, over-responsivity, sensory seeking, and sensory avoiding), their abnormal responses to sensory input can negatively affect their behavior. Environmental sensory input can be modified to improve a student's arousal level by first decreasing environmental sensory input. If this does not bring the student to a quiet, alert state, sensory input can be gradually increased in a socially acceptable manner until a quiet, alert state is achieved.

SENSORY MODULATION STRATEGIES

When a student demonstrates over-responsivity, input within the environment is initially reduced (e.g., by lowering sound volume or using noise-canceling headphones). If a quiet, alert state is not achieved, sensory input is incrementally increased from that lower level in order to enhance learning (e.g., teachers increase the volume of and inflection in their voice) to help students achieve a quiet, alert state. This strategy is particularly useful for students who have both hyper- and hypo-responsivity to sensory input.

The *increase structure and increase response time strategy* prompts staff to structure the environment and pause after speaking, ensuring that the client understands the given directions and expectations and can best respond appropriately. This technique is especially helpful for students with auditory processing challenges. The easiest approach to hypo- or hyper-responsiveness is to reduce the stimulation; then, if a quiet, alert state has not been attained, progressively increase the stimulation in a socially acceptable way. For example, when a teacher recognizes a student is hyper-responsive, they respond by reducing the class noise level and having the student use a study carrel. If the student is still not in a quiet, alert state after the stimuli have been reduced, the teacher would gradually introduce colored lined paper, increase the volume of their voice, and use other strategies to appropriately increase stimulation until the student can achieve a quiet, alert state. Teachers and therapists begin by changing the environment to meet a student's sensory needs, describing the changes that help; but the ultimate goal is for the student to recognize and adapt to their sensory environment in order to independently achieve a quiet, alert state.

Stretching, if done slowly and sustained for ten seconds, can be a mindfulness strategy that reduces the influence of the startle and other primitive reflexes. *Stretch front* is similar to the runner's forward stretch, with one leg in front of the other, but it begins with the back heel up and actively moves opposite symmetrical body extension (e.g., away from a tonic labyrinthine reflex). The child's body weight then sinks downward into both legs, with the back heel lowering as the front knee moves forward over the toes. *Stretch side* is done with one foot facing the toes, laterally aligned with the arch of the opposite foot, and the knee brought forward. During all stretching activities it is important to hold the maximal stretch for ten seconds without bouncing. Teachers and therapists should ensure that the child's position does not bring the knee beyond the toes.

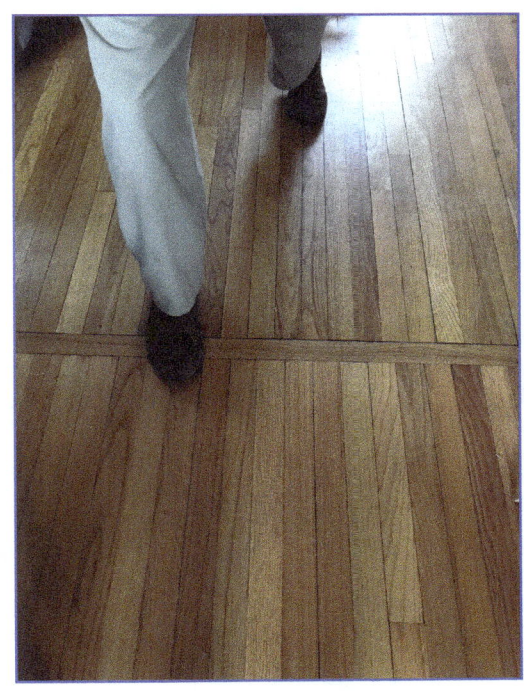

Sensory coaching involves the teacher and therapist helping parents and students discover the best strategies to meet the student's sensory needs. Research suggests that the most affective sensory

33

FAB FUNCTIONALLY ALERT BEHAVIOR STRATEGIES

coaching involves open-ended questions that guide students, such as helping them discover that using hand sanitizer is less upsetting than using soap and water.

Next, graded tactile stimulation activities that can be individualized to provide enriching sensory activities can significantly promote cognitive development in students with intellectual and autism spectrum disorders.[30] By underlining the textures a client is comfortable with, it helps students make progress in processing tactile information. First the client interacts with **beans**, **beans and rice**, then **Theraputty** (progressing from the darkest, most resistant black to the lightest, least resistant yellow), then with **sand**, **Play-Doh**, **water**, **glue**, and **shaving cream**. If the final four textures cannot be tolerated, adaptations are introduced (e.g., using dissolving, rather than liquid, soap; using a glue stick as opposed to glue; using popsicle sticks to apply shaving cream). In order to become desensitized, the client is exposed to the graded textures in a naturalistic setting, using an age-appropriate tactile bin or craft activity.

Self-brushing involves teaching students to brush their arms with a scrub brush, which can be ordered for student use. Self-brushing is taught gradually, beginning with brushing done by the therapist. **Self-brushing** is most often used to replace cutting or other self-injurious behaviors (e.g., scratching, biting, burning). It is usually less satisfying than the self-injurious behavior, so it must be accompanied by strong **reinforcement**. The sensory match strategy is also frequently used with reinforcement to replace aggressive, risky, and unsafe sensory-seeking behaviors.

CHAPTER 3

FAB PRESSURE TOUCH STRATEGIES

This chapter describes FAB Strategies involving moderate and firm touch or massage, which are a small but important portion of the sensory modulation strategies (Figure 3.1). Although these are not used with all students or in all settings, research supports the individualized use of firm and moderate pressure touch as an effective intervention for reducing stress and improving behavior in students with autism spectrum disorder, other developmental disabilities, and sensory modulation challenges.[1] These moderate- and deep-pressure touch strategies are collectively referred to as FAB Pressure Touch strategies. The specific touch selected is individualized to meet the needs of each student. The therapist may select from various touch interventions, including vibration, scrub brushing, pressing with a towel, tapping, and mechanical pressure using a Steamroller Deluxe.

Figure 3.1. FAB PRESSURE TOUCH FORM *Part 1*

Copyright © 2019 by John Pagano, Ph.D., OTR/L, *www.fabstrategies.org*

Client: _____ Date: _____

Therapist: _____ Contact Therapist: _____

Functional Goal: _____

    The FAB Pressure Touch form is an addendum providing a detailed description of the pressure touch strategies listed on the FAB Strategies form. A therapist initially individualizes any pressure touch strategies that can help the client achieve their goals. Before implementation, the therapist ensures that the client doesn't have abrasions, skin problems, osteoporosis, unstable joints, or other conditions that contraindicate pressure touch. The therapist also obtains parental and client consent for using the pressure touch strategies and modifies or discontinues them if the client resists or dislikes the touch.

    Baseline data are collected regarding client goals that research supports could be helped by pressure touch strategies (e.g., decreased anxiety, improved behavior). The therapist can mark which pressure touch strategies to use on the FAB Pressure Touch form and use the letter key to specify the type of pressure touch input: **P**-Deep pressure, **T**-Tapping rapidly, **B**-Brushing, **V**-Vibrating bath brushing, **C**-Joint compression, **Tr**-Traction separating two joints, **M**-Movement described, or **Tow**-pressure applied with a towel. Verbally identifying body parts as they are touched can be helpful for improving body awareness. Accompany or immediately follow pressure touch with functional activities related to goal attainment. Regularly monitor the client for skin abrasions or color changes.

    Once the therapist determines that their implementation of a FAB Pressure Touch strategy is objectively improving the student's behavior, the therapist can offer to show the teacher how to implement the strategy. If further behavioral improvement is seen with the teacher implementing the strategy, the therapist can also teach and reinforce the student for independently using a similar strategy providing comparable sensory input.

    For example, consider a therapist who implements the arm scrub brushing followed by the joint compression strategy with a student daily in the classroom. After two weeks the therapist objectively determines that the student's behavior improves (e.g., the student is now keeping safe hands as evidenced by not hitting peers for an average of two consecutive hours in class, compared with an average of twenty minutes maximum at baseline before implementing the brushing and compression strategy). The therapist would then offer to show the teacher how to do arm brushing followed by joint compression, and describe this procedure in writing using the FAB Strategies and the FAB Pressure Touch form. The therapist would also demonstrate the arm brushing and joint compression strategy on the teacher and coach the teacher in using the strategy with their student.

FAB PRESSURE TOUCH STRATEGIES

After the teacher learns and regularly embeds use of the arm brushing and joint compression strategy as needed in the classroom at least once daily for two weeks, if further behavioral improvement is seen, the therapist would then develop a similar sensory input strategy that the student could do independently. The therapist could teach the student to independently do self-brushing followed by wheelbarrow walking over a therapy ball and reward the student for doing it when they begin feeling angry. After student implementation daily, behavioral progress would then be reassessed.

I. PROGRESSION STRATEGIES (INTRODUCED SEQUENTIALLY):
1. Back Press (apply pressure downward, on each side of the spine) _____
2. Arm Press a) Back of arm fingers to shoulder _____ b) Volar arm to palm _____
3. Arm Compression 10 sec. (shoulder 80°, elbow 85°, wrist 90°) _____
4. Leg Press (down lateral border of thigh & calf, then top of the foot) _____
5. Leg Compression 10 sec. (below knee into hip; above knee down) _____

II. OPTIONS STRATEGIES (ANY ORDER):
1. Head Crown _____
2. Scapula Squeeze _____
3. Shoulders Squeeze _____
4. Shoulders Press _____
5. Spine Roll _____
6. Arm Roll Activity _____
7. Arm Roll _____
8. Arm Wave _____

Reference Video: http://www.youtube.com/watch?v=CTSEd8hWiVI

FAB FUNCTIONALLY ALERT BEHAVIOR STRATEGIES

Figure 3.1. FAB PRESSURE TOUCH FORM *Part 2*

Copyright © 2019 by John Pagano, Ph.D., OTR/L, www.fabstrategies.org

Client: _____ Date: _____

III. BACK TECH: TAP 10X THEN/OR PRESS 10X

  ONE HAND:
- a. Top of the head _____
- b. Back of the head _____
- c. Back of the neck (gently contouring) _____
- d. Down the spine _____

  TWO HANDS:
- a. Back of the thighs _____
- b. Back of the calves _____
- c. Back of the feet _____
  Reference Video: https://www.youtube.com/watch?v=MviTjCz7–38

IV. TAP SELF: EAR TO PALM _____
- a. Tap back of the hand
- b. Tap up the arm
- c. Tap on the shoulder
- d. Tap on the neck
- e. Tap around ear
- f. Tap on the neck (gently contouring)
- g. Turn palm up and tap down the arm to the palm

V. PRESS SELF: EAR TO PALM _____
- a. Press on the back of the hand
- b. Press up the arm
- c. Press on the shoulder
- d. Press on the neck
- e. Press on the ear
- f. Press on the neck
- g. Press on shoulder
- h. Turn palm up and press down the arm to the palm

FAB PRESSURE TOUCH STRATEGIES

VI. TAP SELF: HEAD TO FEET
   a. Tap the top of head
   b. Tap the back of the head
   c. Tap the back of the neck (gently contouring)
   d. Tap progressively down the sides of the trunk
   e. Tap progressively down the sides of the legs

VII. PRESS SELF: HEAD TO FEET
   a. Press the top of head
   b. Press the back of the head
   c. Press the back of the neck (gently contouring)
   d. Press progressively down the sides of the trunk
   e. Press progressively down the sides of the legs

References:

www6.miami.edu/touch-research   www.qsti.org

FAB FUNCTIONALLY ALERT BEHAVIOR STRATEGIES

Touch Strategies Listed on the FAB Forms

Touch vibration provides alerting proprioceptive and tactile sensations that promote body awareness. **Touch vibration** can be provided with a vibrating bath brush (e.g., Jiggle Gator), rather than through massage, making it a useful alternative to massage for many teachers, nurses, mental health therapists, and other professionals who are uncomfortable with providing hands-on touch. Touch vibration can be helpful for students with sensory discrimination disorders by giving them increased awareness of their body. It is also often a helpful alternative for students who engage in self-harm by cutting themselves or who are not respecting physical boundaries because they are craving touch.

Touch vibration for body awareness can be useful in conjunction with self-touch (see Figure 6.2 on P. 85, FAB Strategies Pre-K & Kindergarten form, Section B). Touch vibration is best introduced sequentially with **Touch vibration back**, **Touch vibration arms** (initially on the back of the arm then, if desired, on the surface of the palm), and finally **Touch vibration body** on the hands, feet, and face, if needed.

Touch vibration back is done first, providing vibration on each side of the back, but not crossing the spine initially. Later, back vibration can be provided across the spine as tolerated. **Touch vibration arms** is done from proximal to distal, beginning at the shoulder and proceeding to the fingertips. **Touch vibration body** is a useful game for improving body awareness and tactile discrimination; with children older than seven, the concepts of right and left may be added. It can be done initially with their eyes closed then with their eyes open. If an error is made—for example, if a client with their eyes closed guesses elbow when touched on the ankle—simply offer basic choices, such as, "Is it your ankle or your nose?"

Light touch and tapping strategies are used to improve body awareness and alertness and to decrease experiences of pain. They are more likely than deep-pressure touch to result in arousal, and an increase in arousal level is possible. It is important to also provide students with many light-

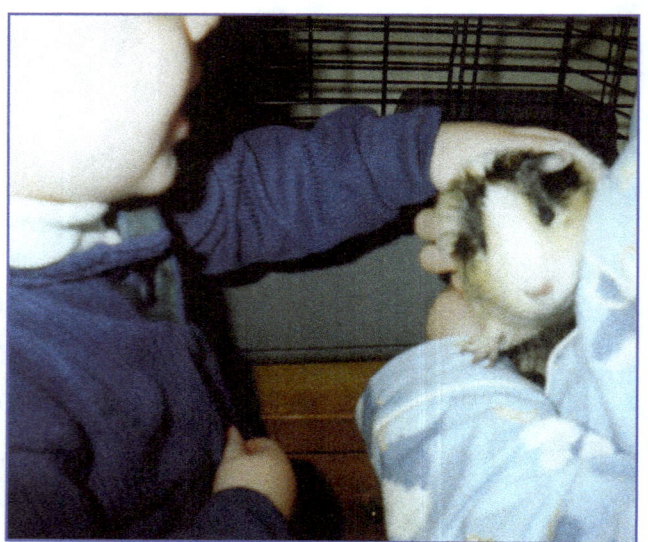

touch opportunities through typical occupational experiences such as caring for classroom pets.

A therapist or peer can introduce light-touch using the X Marks the Spot game. The X Marks the Spot game includes the **back X** in which the therapist "draws" an X with their fist on the student's back. This provides light-touch and gives the student increased awareness of their back. The **back crawl** strategy is a second light-touch strategy providing the student with an increased awareness of their back. To do the **back crawl**, the therapist alternately uses their

FAB PRESSURE TOUCH STRATEGIES

knuckles on opposite sides of the student's spine to move sequentially up their back while saying "creepy crawlies up your back."

In the *egghead strategy* the therapist, after getting the student's permission, pretends to crack an egg on their head. The *egghead strategy* is done by the therapist making a fist with one hand, pressing down forcefully on their fist with their opposite hand, then moving the fingers of both their hands simultaneously downward on the two sides of the student's head. The therapist's movements provide light-touch input that gives increased awareness to the student's head, orienting the student through touch to the top of their body.

The **foot input** strategy involves pressing down on the ankle or vibrating the feet to provide awareness of the feet and help the student feel stable. While doing this the therapist can simultaneously provide the verbal prompts "make your feet steady and stable like the roots of a tree." Awareness of the head through the **egghead** and foot through the **foot input** strategy promotes basic body awareness by orienting the student to the top and bottom of their body.

Tap-press self involves two self-touch strategies that promote body awareness and can act as a sensory replacement for self-cutting or scratching. Revised from Tui Na massage for children with autism spectrum disorders, Tap-press self can be done through two sequences involving pressing and tapping. **Tap-press self: Ear to arm** (see P. 38 IV. & V.) involves first tapping around the ear with a claw hand, then using an open hand to tap on the neck, proceeding down the arm to the palm. Next, the client presses their ear and neck, continuing to press. **Tap-press self: Head to feet** (see P. 39, VI. VII.) involves self-pressing or tapping followed by pressing on the top of the head, back of the head, back of the neck, and down the sides, from below the arms to the ankles, with both hands.

Several FAB Pressure Touch strategies are listed on the FAB Trigger & Coping form. A more detailed explanation of these strategies as well as additional strategies can be found on the FAB Pressure Touch form. The FAB Pressure Touch form (see PP. 36–39) can be added as an addenum to the FAB Strategies form. All of these strategies are to be developed by a trained therapist and then taught to other team members.

FAB Pressure Touch strategies reduce anxiety, promote communication, and improve behavior in clients with behavioral and developmental challenges. FAB Pressure Touch strategies are a unique approach synthesizing evidence-based massage, bodywork, and scrub brushing strategies. They help children, adolescents, and adults who have behavioral, psychiatric, sensory processing, trauma history, and developmental challenges.

Distinct from commonly used therapeutic brushing, massage, and bodywork "sensory stimulation" strategies, FAB Pressure Touch strategies are individualized to achieve specific therapeutic goals. They are a goal-directed component of a comprehensive FAB strategies intervention addressing problematic hypo-responsiveness, hyper-responsiveness, anxiety, social skills, behavioral challenges, and developmental challenges.

FAB FUNCTIONALLY ALERT BEHAVIOR STRATEGIES

Trained occupational, physical, speech/language, and mental health therapists develop individual FAB Pressure Touch strategies for each student to help achieve the student's functional behavioral goals. Goals may include increased attention span, seated attention, communication skills, social interactions, and use of safe hands (e.g., decreased physical aggression). Therapists can teach the individualized FAB Pressure Touch strategies to parents, teachers, and other team members embedded in the client's daily routine. Once implementation of the FAB Pressure Touch strategies is found to improve behavior, clients are taught and reinforced for independently engaging in sensory behavioral strategies providing equivalent pressure touch and resistance exercise input.

FAB Pressure Touch strategies include the Head crown, Shoulder squeeze, Spine roll, Back Tech tap, Back Tech press, touch on the back, as well as touch and joint compression through the arms, legs, and feet. The FAB Pressure Touch Strategies form can be attached to the FAB Strategies form to provide more detailed touch strategies. In my sensory behavioral strategies workshops for therapists and teachers, I teach goal-directed development and implementation of FAB Pressure Touch strategies. Afterward, many teachers report that intermittently using the shoulder press strategy increases the student's attention span and frustration tolerance during seated writing activities.

The first line of the Pagano FAB Pressure Touch strategies listed on the Sensory Behavioral Strategies to Promote Self-control form lists optional strategies that can be applied individually or in any order to reduce stress, enhance relationships, and contribute to functional skills. All of the options on the first line involve contouring the therapist's hands to the shape of the client's body, then gradually increasing the touch to very deep pressure, as tolerated. The **head crown strategy** involves the therapist applying deep pressure with their hands, which are contoured to the shape of the child's head. The therapist applies pressure with open hands on both sides of the child's head for ten seconds, then on the front and back of the head for ten seconds.

The **head crown strategy** is useful for reducing anxiety and reinforcing desirable behavior. This **strategy** can also be embedded in the daily routine as an antecedent sensory match strategy and non-contingent reinforcement to promote acceptance of hair washing, cutting, or braiding by clients with touch defensiveness. As with all FAB Pressure Touch strategies, it begins with contouring, whereby the therapist's hands form around the body part like sinking into mud, then gradually providing deep pressure. In addition, it can be used as an antecedent sensory match strategy and non-contingent reinforcement for helping clients with tactile-seeking behaviors; in this case it can act as a replacement behavior for self-injurious head banging. Many therapists, teachers, and parents report that using the head crown strategy helps calm students who are becoming frustrated while doing school or homework and improved the children's ability to tolerate having their hair brushed without complaining of discomfort.

The **shoulder squeeze** strategy involves forceful pressure through both shoulders for ten seconds, with the force applied three-dimensionally, diagonally inward and downward, through the shoulders toward the center of the trunk. The **shoulders press** strategy provides pressure directly down through the trunk. Pressure is applied three-dimensionally, inward and downward through the trunk region. All three FAB Pressure Touch strategies can be done while the client is seated or standing and are embedded into their functional activities. The *scapula squeeze* strategy involves ten seconds of pressure that is applied through a front-to-back pancaking motion, which applies pressure to and reduces muscle tone in the shoulder blades. The **arm roll strategy** often follows the *scapula squeeze* strategy to increase body awareness and motor planning. The therapist rolls the student's upper arm toward a position with the hand open and the thumb positioned laterally. Next, a handshake position is used, with a slight outward pull to provide traction, and the arm is moved toward a palm-up position with the hand open.

The **spine roll** strategy can be done with the child seated but is best applied when the child lies prone; this enables greater pressure to be applied. The therapist applies pressure with one hand that they first slide from just below the child's neck to the lower spine. When that hand reaches the lower spine, the therapist applies pressure with the opposite hand, beginning below the neck, before the lower hand is removed and the progression continues. This strategy applies continuous pressure to promote parasympathetic calming.

The *arm roll activity* strategy is an effective movement break that is listed only on the FAB Pressure Touch Strategy addendum but can be added to the FAB Strategy to Promote Self-control sheet. It can be done individually and in group and whole-class environments. The adult models and describes one hand moving up and out, like an imaginary super-powerful helium balloon, and raises their arm as high as possible, then passively drops the arm, representing the balloon popping. The arm must fall passively and not be thrown downward. This strategy enables the child to experience traction at the shoulder as the balloon rises, followed by passive traction down as the arm falls due to the force of gravity. Next, imagining that one arm is a fishing line and the hand is the sinker, the child moves toward a hands-open position with the thumb lateral. As the hands move, the child sequentially visualizes the thumb, index finger, middle finger, ring finger, and pinky. Next, the child tries to visualize all of the joints in the hand. Finally, the child tries to feel the back of the arm, then stops.

The **arm wave** strategy is another option for increasing body awareness and motor planning. The client grasps the dorsal surface of the hand between the knuckles of the index and middle and the middle and ring fingers, then shakes the hand vertically as the hand is slowly raised, then lowered.

FAB Pressure Touch involves deep pressure with a scrub brush, vibrating bath brush, pressure from the therapist's hand, or a scratchy towel. **FAB Pressure Touch** using a scrub brush is also referred to as *FAB Brushing*, to clarify that it is different from the Wilbarger Brushing Protocol (deep pressure and proprioceptive technique). FAB Brushing differs from the Wilbarger Protocol, but two case studies showed that both the FAB and Wilbarger forms of deep-pressure brushing significantly improved occupational performance in two five-year-old students with autism spectrum disorder.[2]

FAB FUNCTIONALLY ALERT BEHAVIOR STRATEGIES

FAB Pressure Touch differs from the Wilbarger Brushing Protocol in that the therapist individualizes it and embeds it in the class or home routine, and no minimal amount of time is necessary, as described in part I of the FAB Pressure Touch form, "Progression Strategies" (see Figure 3.1). FAB Pressure Touch is usually introduced sequentially, although not all of the strategies need to be completed. Firm deep pressure is used most often, although some children prefer moderate pressure. Light pressure is usually avoided on the arms because it is not perceived as calming by most students. Pressure touch should be stopped immediately if the student resists; it can be reoffered later. The sequential progression of touch occurs on the back, then on the arms, legs, and feet. Pressure begins on the least sensitive body areas and proceeds as needed to the most sensitive. First, the child is touched with deep pressure on each side of the spinal column without crossing the midline. Research has shown that just ten minutes of back massage significantly improves behavior in adolescents with mental health challenges.[3]

Next, pressure is applied on the back dorsal surface of each arm, progressing from the fingertips to the shoulder. Touch pressure is then given through the arms by giving input to the many pressure receptors located around the joints; this promotes a calm, alert state.

Joint compression provides body awareness and calming. Several joint compression activities are included on the FAB Pressure Touch Strategies form. Joint compression creates the same effect that is achieved by hugging or holding a child to calm them. In this same way, when students wheelbarrow walk or do isometrics, they are independently providing themselves with calming joint compression input.

FAB Pressure Touch back is introduced first because the back is usually the least sensitive area. The touch moves gradually from the shoulders toward the waist on one side of the spine, then the other, initially avoiding movement across the spine. **FAB Pressure Touch back** is used until the client is comfortable with it. **FAB Pressure Touch arm** is done next, with deep pressure on the dorsal surface (back) of the arm, initially proceeding from the fingertips to the shoulder. After FAB Pressure Touch arm is completed, joint compression is done for ten seconds at each shoulder, elbow, and wrist. Ensure good joint alignment; in particular, the wrist should be straight (e.g., not flexed, extended, or in radial or ulnar deviation).

FAB Pressure Touch arm is consistently followed by joint compression to provide relaxing pressure that can be easily tolerated. **Arm traction** is done at a separate time to increase body awareness, frequently after or accompanying the arm roll or arm shake movements. **Arm roll** is a rolling movement of the arm toward a hand position with the palm up and the thumb lateral. The **arm shake** is a vertical shaking of the arm while the shoulder moves first upward into full flexion, then into full extension. The **arm roll** and **arm shake** are done gently and accompanied by or followed by arm traction; they are designed to increase body awareness.

My clinical experience strongly suggests that to maximally calm and promote appropriate behavior in students with complex behavioral strategies, arm brushing should be followed by ten consecutive seconds of joint compression provided at the shoulder, elbow, and wrist. Further, it appears most effective for calming students to provide joint compression with the shoulder in 80 degrees of abduction, the elbow in 80 degrees of extension, and the wrist straight so it is at a 90-degree angle.

Therapists can use the FAB Pressure Touch form (Figure 3.1) both as a reference and to develop individualized programs that teachers and parents can implement. It is important for therapists to determine the most effective touch strategies before assigning them as part of a home program. It is also helpful to embed the touch strategies in the student's school or home routine. Touch strategies should be taught to teachers or parents before they are assigned as part of a home program.

For children who frequently walk on their toes or demonstrate other potentially problematic behaviors that suggest atypical sensory perception of the feet (e.g., sitting with the chair legs pressing on their feet or refusing to wear socks and shoes), it can be helpful to include brushing of the leg and foot followed by joint compression. Brushing and compression followed by stretching of the ankle can promote sensory awareness and mobility of the legs and feet that may help the student avoid consistent toe walking and the possible development of future ankle joint problems. Stretching of the ankle can be done by the therapist to promote typical joint mobility. Pressure to the legs is initially applied on the lateral border of the thigh, then on the lateral border of the calf, and finally the dorsal surface (top) of the foot. After pressure is put on the leg joints, compression is applied. Provide joint compression to the hip and ankle with the student sitting so the knee and ankle are in 90 degrees of flexion with the foot supported on the floor. First, support the student at the pelvis and hold him below the knee, pressing into the hip for ten seconds. Next, hold above the knee and press the foot downward into the floor for ten seconds. If toe walking makes tight hamstrings a concern, roll the supported foot then dorsiflex and elongate the ankle.

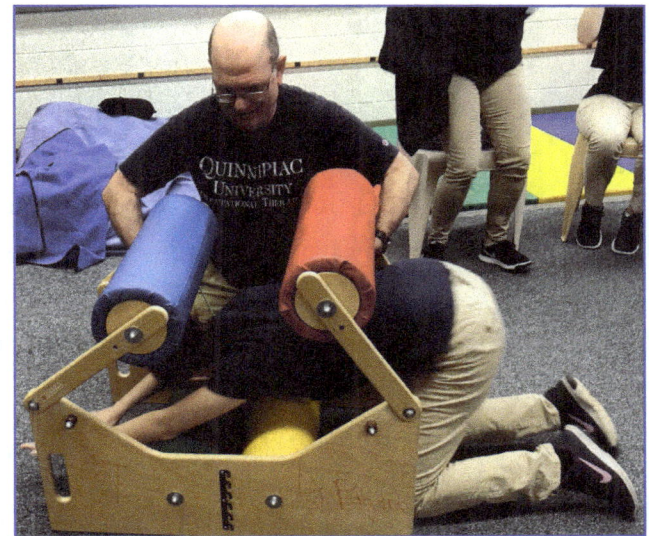

The **Steamroller Deluxe** is a commercial product that provides mechanical deep-pressure support. The therapist helps the student get into the Steamroller Deluxe and invites them to stay for up to ten minutes while playing with a toy. This can be very calming and help decrease aggressive and self-injurious behaviors. It is important for the therapist to monitor the student's chest to ensure the student is breathing comfortably. The student should get out immediately if they experience any discomfort.

A **mat sandwich** is a strategy in which the therapist provides deep pressure on the student by pressing on the student's body with a mat. The therapist consistently monitors the mat sandwich to be sure that the student is breathing comfortably; the position can be held up to five minutes. The student controls the pressure by constantly indicating whether they want more pressure, less pressure, or the mat taken off.

Roll therapy ball on involves firmly pressing down and rolling a therapy ball over the student's back. **Roll therapy ball on-Core progression** involves pressing a therapy ball on a client's body in a specific developmental sequence to improve body awareness. First, downward pressure is applied on the center of the client's back (opposite the navel) for three minutes. The firm pressure promotes the student's awareness of their back (e.g., where the ball is pressing). The second developmental movement involves rolling the ball over the arms three times before returning to center, then rolling the therapy ball over the legs three times before returning to center. These movements help orient the student to the top and bottom of their body.

The third developmental progression involves rolling the therapy ball over the right arm and leg three times then returning to center, then rolling the ball over the left arm and leg three times. The right and left side movements are to provide the student with awareness to the two sides of their body. A treatment video of Roll therapy ball on-Core progression is available at https://www.youtube.com/watch?v=LCD9JeFviKY.

The fourth and most advanced developmental progression that can be included in Roll therapy ball on-Core progression involves providing sensory awareness of the relationship between the opposing arm and leg of the body used in reciprocal movements such as walking. This fourth progression is done by rolling the therapy ball over the right arm and moving it diagonally across the center of the body to roll over the left leg. This movement of rolling the therapy ball over the right arm and left leg is repeated two more times. Following this, the ball is rolled to center, then rolled over the left arm and diagonally to the right leg, with this movement repeated two more times before returning to center. Roll therapy ball on-Core progression is concluded by returning to center and pressing down on the therapy ball at center for three minutes.

Back tech (see section III., P. 38) is an adaptation based on QiGong Sensory Treatment (QST)[4] that when used in its entirety improves behavior, sensory modulation, and communication skills in preschool through fifth-grade students with autism spectrum disorder,[5,6] including both those with hyposensitivity and those with hypersensitivity to touch.[7] Most of the research and reviews supporting massage for improving behavior involve QST or Thai massage using acupressure points that normalize hypo-responsive and hyper-responsive reactions of students with autism spectrum disorder.[8] Research indicates that children with less severe ASD showed significantly better results with only parental massage, whereas those with more severe ASD did significantly better given both massage by both a therapist and a parent.[9]

Students are given the opportunity to receive either vigorous tapping or slow, deep-pressing sensory input. I have observed clinically that most students prefer only pressing input, whereas students

FAB PRESSURE TOUCH STRATEGIES

who have hypotonicity and aggressive behavior usually select the tapping and the pressing input. If students select both inputs, then tapping is done ten times followed by pressing ten times. This involves sequentially tapping or pressing on a student who is lying on his stomach: first with one hand on top of the head, then the back of the head, the back of the neck, down the spine; then both hands are used simultaneously to provide input on both thighs, calves, and feet.

All the supported sitting on therapy ball movements (see P. 79, last row in Section B) are done with the child sitting as independently as possible on the therapy ball with the therapist adding more support prior to moving the student. First, **supported sitting on therapy ball forward & back** is done by having the student sit on the therapy ball, holding the student at the pelvis, with their permission, and moving the ball **Forward & back** three times. Next **supported sitting on therapy ball Up & down** is done with the student sitting on the therapy ball and the therapist holding around the student's shoulders. The therapist presses downward on the shoulders then allows the ball to rebound, moving the student back up three times. If the student is able to tolerate the first two movements, the therapist can proceed to **supported sitting on therapy ball sides**. The therapist supports the child in sitting by holding them at the pelvis and moving them side to side, facilitating a lateral righting reaction (e.g., the therapist provides movement to the right, and the student flexes their head and trunk laterally to the left to maintain their balance).

Supported sitting on a therapy ball mindful clock combines all the previously mentioned **supported sitting on a therapy ball** activities described above (e.g., forward and back, down and up, then side to side). Each is done while saying "tic-toc, like a clock, till we find our center." **Supported sitting on a therapy ball mindful clock** is intentionally similar to the **mindful clock sitting** and **mindful clock standing** strategies described in the previous chapter. **Mindful clock sitting** and **mindful clock standing** can be easily done in classroom settings, enabling therapists and teachers to work collaboratively so students who have special needs can do similar activities in their mainstream classrooms and therapy sessions.

FAB Strategies enable therapists and teachers to provide consistent strategies for students with complex behavior challenges in the classroom, small groups, and individual therapy settings. The environmental adaptation and sensory modulation strategies presented in previous chapters provide the foundation for the FAB Pressure Touch Strategies described in this chapter. The positive behavior support strategies presented in the next chapter will complement and reinforce the strategies we have already learned.

A video of an intervention session by the author demonstrating the FAB Pressure Touch Strategies being done with a preschooler who has autism spectrum disorder and behavioral challenges is available online at https://www.youtube.com/watch?v=CTSEd8hWiVI.

It is essential before doing the FAB Pressure Touch strategies to always be sure that there are no bone or joint contraindications and that breathing is never compromised. Also, touch is never done

FAB FUNCTIONALLY ALERT BEHAVIOR STRATEGIES

without the permission of the student and their parents and is immediately discontinued if the student asks the therapist to stop or complains of any discomfort.

It is important to remember that all of the FAB Pressure Touch strategies comprise a small component of the sensory modulation strategies section of the FAB Strategies form. The FAB Pressure Touch strategies are sometimes not included in a student's intervention, such as in instances where a student has a history of PTSD, medical contraindications, or simply dislikes touch. However, the FAB Pressure Touch strategies are described in detail because they are an important component of treatment for some students with complex behavioral challenges, as these interventions can be extremely helpful for some students with severe developmental disabilities and aggressive behavior.

The FAB Pressure Touch strategies should be selected and used only by or under the direction of trained occupational, physical, and speech/language therapists. Speech/language pathologists have successfully used and taught many of the FAB Pressure Touch strategies to reduce anxiety, improve behavior, and promote motor planning skills for improved functional communication. However, each speech/language pathologist must determine which FAB Pressure Touch strategies they are comfortable doing and ensure they are consistent with their scope of practice.

CHAPTER 4

POSITIVE BEHAVIOR SUPPORT STRATEGIES

Positive behavior support strategies are largely based on sensory integration theory integrated with pivotal response training (PRT), the Promoting Alternative THinking Strategies (PATHS), Second Step, and Devereux Early Childhood Assessment (DECA) program. PRT is an applied behavioral analysis method developed by an expert behaviorist and speech/language pathologist. PRT uses applied behavioral analysis to developmentally promote motivation, generalization, and social interaction. PATHS, Second Step, and the DECA, are positive behavioral support programs used widely in schools with typical students to improve their social skills and behavior. Through integrating sensory integration and behavioral programs, the positive behavior support section provides strategies that use sensory integration principles to improve behavior.

FAB Strategies are unique in their multidisciplinary integration of positive behavioral support with sensory-based interventions. Because sensory-based interventions motivate most students, combining them with behavioral strategies increases the likelihood that students will do them. Hitting, punching, and self-injurious behaviors reflect a lack of inhibitory motor control. Sensory and behavioral strategies can be combined to teach students self-control, enabling them to be aware of their environmental and body triggers, and to implement sensory coping strategies in order to avoid inappropriate behavior.

Clinical reasoning is used to develop an individualized approach that integrates PRT, positive behavioral support, as well as the environmental adaptation, sensory modulation, mindfulness, and touch strategies described in the preceding chapters. Because children with complex behavioral challenges frequently also have developmental and mental health diagnoses, an understanding of these challenges and their significantly increased likelihood of resulting in neurological differences makes a flexible clinical reasoning approach much more beneficial than rigid discipline.

Clinical reasoning includes the previously mentioned strategies of individual developmental assessment and consistent use of a trauma-informed approach. For example, students who have experienced physical abuse during childhood (which school therapists and teachers may be unaware of) are significantly more likely to have a small orbitofrontal lobe, which is directly linked to academic, behavioral, and social skill difficulties.[1] Students who have diagnoses of depression or bipolar, anxiety, and autism spectrum disorders (which teachers may also be unaware of) are more sensitive to facial responses because of increased neurological activation of the amygdala. Awareness of these differences may enable therapists and teachers to consistently remove these students from interactions with classmates and to maintain a calm facial expression before students begin to have a tantrum, which helps to minimize the risk of the student becoming aggressive.[2]

Pivotal Response Training

FAB Strategies of preferred tasks, choices, priming, and reinforce attempts are all based on Pivotal Response Training (PRT), which is a proven intervention that uses applied behavioral analysis to developmentally promote motivation, behavioral self-regulation, generalization, and communication in students with developmental and autism spectrum disorders (ASD). It is especially clinically relevant for students with complex behavioral challenges, because behavioral skills cannot be addressed without simultaneously improving motivation and behavioral self-regulation.[3]

PRT is an especially useful intervention for therapists and teachers because it is practically applicable when addressing complex behavioral challenges in students of various ages, with various developmental disabilities and diagnoses, and in various settings. It includes family members, teachers, and occupational, speech/language, and mental health therapists in the intervention and encourages the use of engaging sensory activities in the classroom environment. Research supports the use of PRT both individually and in groups for preschool through third grade; it increases engagement among these students and can be used by special education teachers to increase engagement and reduce the number of disruptions.[4]

Research supports that the use of PRT with preschoolers who had autism spectrum disorder significantly improved their social communication.[5] This same research also found neurological changes, such that the preschoolers with baseline hypo-reactivity showed increased activation of the neural reward system, whereas those with initial hyperactivity and behavioral control difficulties showed decreased activation of the subcortical neural regions that stimulate the cortex.[5]

The desensitization and self-management strategies are PRT interventions that help students with developmental and behavioral challenges learn to independently modify their behavior to respond in a socially acceptable way to the sensory challenges of their natural environment.[6] The **ask permission to kid** and **ask permission to touch others** strategies also are used to teach students to generalize their behavior to the school environment. The desensitization and self-management strategies are adapted from the PRT approach to help students with developmental and behavioral challenges to generalize their behavior to the sensory challenges within and social needs of the natural environment.[6]

Three strategies use playful prompts in naturalistic school settings to promote appropriate social skills. The first two are reminders to **ask permission to kid** and **ask permission to touch** others; these ensure that kidding and touching are consistent with social skills appropriate for school.

The third self-regulation strategy, **prompt filter speech**, involves the teacher or therapist motioning as though they are hitting themselves in the head while saying "that comment should have stayed in your head." These strategies can be humorously used in specific situations to help students respect interpersonal boundaries. A helpful way of teaching **prompt filter speech** is to review mindfulness guidelines and make sure they are all answered with "yes" before speaking: "Is it true? Is it kind? Is it necessary?"[7]

Teachers and therapists can repeatedly model these behaviors by asking students for permission to kid with them and to touch them, and noting when the student has inappropriately said something they should have "kept in their head" and not said. As a therapist who frequently uses massage and who is of Italian ancestry, I always model asking permission before kidding with or touching others, and I jokingly remind and strongly reinforce clients for following these same practices. Along with using these three playful prompts, it is extremely important to "catch" and reinforce students for demonstrating appropriate boundaries around kidding, touching, and speaking to others.

The **invite** strategy involves respectfully asking students to do things but not coercing them. It is a trauma-informed care strategy that avoids conflicts with students that may occur when they are "forced" to do things. **Invite** is done through simple statements such as, "You can close your eyes to do the breathing exercises if you would like. I'm going to keep mine open to keep you safe." The invite strategy also involves letting students choose to sit quietly and not participate in exercises or activities as long as they don't distract classmates.

The **will like you** trauma-informed strategy involves consistently assuring students that "[the therapist or teacher] like[s] you and **will like you** regardless of your behavior." The **will like you** strategy confirms that teachers and therapists will always like the student no matter what behavior they exhibit, although the teachers and therapists will use rewards and punishment to ensure that the student learns behaviors that will make them successful in the future. While particularly useful for students with attachment and post-traumatic stress disorders, this strategy shows respect for all students and helps avoid power struggles.

Social role-playing can be done individually or with small groups of students. It is useful for discussing, reviewing, and practicing social situations. **Social role-playing** can help students practice a variety of social situations, such as how close to stand to others in social situations and how to ask to join peers in a game; it can also help them model and guess each other's feelings. While social role-playing can be done individually, it is also presented as a component of a social skills group.

FAB FUNCTIONALLY ALERT BEHAVIOR STRATEGIES

Participation in a social skills group that applies the PEERS Curriculum is a proven strategy for improving social skills in students with ASD.[8] Research demonstrates the effectiveness of a social skills group curriculum for students with typical intellectual ability: It not only significantly improves functional social skills, but also significantly increases the left hemisphere-dominant asymmetry associated with typical students, and it provides greater motivation and helps to create a more positive affect.[9] I use this social skills curriculum for students with mental health and intellectual disabilities, and I emphasize portions of the curriculum that teach effective strategies for dealing with bullies.

While the effectiveness of social skills groups using the PEERS Curriculum was studied only in students with ASD and typical intelligence, approximately 70 percent of children with ASD have a comorbid sensory modulation or mental health disorder (e.g., social anxiety, attention deficit hyperactivity disorder [ADHD], oppositional defiant disorder).[10] I adapted the PEERS Curriculum social skills group for special populations and have been using it with clinical success for over three years. This social skills group for special populations includes students who have ASD as well as intellectual, sensory modulation, and mental health disorders.

I made several modifications when conducting the social skills group for special populations. First, it is helpful for special populations to have at least two leaders for social skills groups of two to eight students, including some with typical intelligence and compliant behavior but who are extremely shy. Research and clinical experience support adding a snack time, alternating movement and seated activities, incorporating sensory coping strategies to modulate the students' arousal level, minimizing distractions (e.g., closing the window shades), and teaching sensory coping strategies.[11]

My social skills group for special populations covers half of the information in the typical PEERS Curriculum to allow for more activities and snack time. I cover bullying as well; and when time is limited, I find it particularly useful to teach students to manage online, verbal, and physical bullying with the **bully proof strategy**. This strategy uses a PEERS Curriculum social skills group to teach groups of students with ASDs to avoid verbal and physical bullying. Through role-playing and interactions, students are taught to differentiate a bully who verbally teases from a physical bully. To deal with a teasing bully, students are taught to make a brief verbal comeback (e.g., "So what?" "Anyway," or "Who cares?") then walk away. To deal with a physically aggressive bully, students learn not to police the bully, make friends with the bully, respond to the bully with teasing comebacks, or call attention to themselves around the bully. Instead, they are taught to hang around with other people, avoid the bully, stay near an adult when the bully is present, and tell a teacher if the bully is hurting someone, but request that the teacher not tell the bully who told.

In the social skills group for special populations I have added the **switch hands toss** strategy to integrate movement with the verbal expression of feelings. This strategy is a useful sensory variation for teaching social skills to students with more severe behavioral challenges. The **switch hands toss** strategy involves students passing a beanbag while expressing their **favorite** sport, color, ice cream,

POSITIVE BEHAVIOR SUPPORT STRATEGIES

sports team, vacation place, coping strategy, quality when choosing a friend, quality that makes someone a good friend, and other categories. If a student is willing to go first, he or she can pick a category to begin the game. *Guess the feeling* involves a student acting out a feeling using their face and body; the student who catches the beanbag must try to identify the feeling being depicted. The *I feel* strategy involves students stating how they currently feel.

The most challenging **switch hands toss** strategy is the *I message*. An "I message" is a statement in which a student describes an action that others do, how the student feels when that action occurs, and the behavior the student wants others to do instead. The student says, "When people _____, I feel _____, so _____." Here's a positive example: "When people say hi to me, I feel happy, so please say 'hi' when you see me." An example of a complaint is, "When people call me 'Shortie,' I feel angry, so please call me 'John.'" Combining movement with the understanding and expression of feelings makes it a fun game and encourages participation.

Redirection is a useful strategy for students at a chrononological or developmental age of five years or younger. It involves interrupting negative or innapropriate behavior by changing the subject or activity. *Redirection to a favorite activity* can be particularly useful for avoiding aggression if used when students begin to show environmental triggers (e.g., appearing tired) and body triggers (e.g., hand fisting) they should avoid. Try verbal redirection first to change the subject or activity in order to interrupt inappropriate behavior. If verbal redirection is unsuccessful, attempt to physically coax the student toward an alternative activity.[12]

The **breaks** strategy involves the strategic use of developmentally appropriate music, mindfulness, and movement activities to promote appropriate classroom behavior and learning. Before class music and movement breaks, remind the student: "Don't touch anybody, don't touch anything, and get back to work as soon as the break is over so we can do it again tomorrow." **Breaks** are useful to interrupt prolonged sitting, promote body awareness, and as a pre-correction strategy; to consolidate learning between subjects; and to provide aerobic exercise that facilitates learning.

Sensory and movement **breaks** are useful for enabling students with ASD and other developmental disabilities to successfully participate in social skill and cognitive behavioral therapy by giving these students opportunities for movement and sensory activities that can keep them engaged. Adapting social skill and cognitive behavioral therapy sessions to make them engaging and fun often requires collaboration between occupational, speech/language, and mental health therapists, as well as regular and special education teachers. In one case, adapting a cognitive behavioral therapy intervention by providing sensory breaks enabled the intervention to significantly reduce anxiety in students with ASDs.[13]

The **breaks** strategy facilitates inclusion and helps all students learn self-control and attention skills. The strategies benefit typical children but are particularly valuable for children with complex developmental and self-control challenges (including ADHD and ASDs), significantly improving behavior and on-task attention in school. Children with developmental and self-control challenges frequently lose recess privileges because of behavioral difficulties during or after large group physical activities. Discipline problems can be significantly reduced by initially limiting group size, increasing structure, and providing extra movement breaks as a reward for returning to academic effort immediately after physical activities.

Self-management refers to independently monitoring and rewarding improvement in one's own behavior. Research indicates that **self-management** can significantly improve the social skills of students with ASDs.[6] It is important to ensure that a student has learned the skill (e.g., the appropriate way to greet people) before beginning the self-management strategy in order to increase their use of it in their natural environment. The **self-management** strategy includes determining the target behavior (the goal), gathering all the necessary materials, developing a reward system, recording progress, and monitoring success. Therapists and teachers initially review the student's progress and reward them when they attain a goal. Eventually, the behavior becomes automatic and the rewards are faded out.

The **tolerance for delay** strategy helps students gradually improve their frustration tolerance skills by learning to wait for attention or tangible items. For example, consider a student who screams when they are not given individual attention every ten seconds. The teacher gives the student a time delay signal at eight seconds, such as, "I'll be right there." If the student goes eleven seconds without screaming, they are rewarded. Another example is a student who does only ten math problems before misbehaving to escape work. This student would be given a delay signal such as, "Do just one more problem," and they would receive a reward if they achieve this.

Tolerance for delay is especially useful for students who are entering preschool or kindergarten with limited school experience, or who are transitioning from a special education class with a 4-to-1 student-teacher ratio to a regular class with thirty students and one teacher. Waiting and other frustration tolerance skills are learned gradually. **Tolerance for delay** allows therapists and teachers to reinforce students for gradual improvement in their ability to wait for attention.

The **conditioned calm recall** strategy is a unique FAB Strategy that uses classical conditioning to decrease aggression in children who have severe developmental disabilities. Conditioned calm recall involves repeatedly pairing an unconditional stimulus (e.g., specific deep-pressure touch, movement, or music activity) that calms the student through the use of a specific conditioned stimulus (e.g., a lavender-scented ball). During the student's daily routine (e.g., occupational, physical, speech, or mental health therapy interventions), the conditioned stimulus is repeatedly paired with the unconditional calming stimulus. This repeated pairing of the conditioned stimulus with a state of relaxation eventually teaches the student to relax when they receive the conditioned stimulus.

When the student is exposed later to environmental triggers (e.g., school tasks) or shows body triggers (e.g., crying or body tensing), the conditioned stimulus is provided to calm the student, and they are immediately reinforced for avoiding aggression. This teaches nonverbal, developmentally

POSITIVE BEHAVIOR SUPPORT STRATEGIES

disabled children to behave less aggressively. The conditioned stimulus promotes relaxation so the child can be reinforced for reduced aggression.

Sensory matching is useful with students who are found by the Questions About Behavioral Function (QABF) assessment to be engaging in self-injurious behaviors primarily for "nonsocial" (e.g., automatic sensory) reinforcement. Sensory matching requires the therapist to figure out the sensory input the student receives from the inappropriate behavior. Next, using a preference assessment, the therapist offers several more appropriate activities that seem to provide matching sensory input. The preferred sensory matching activity is offered as non-contingent reinforcement (e.g., it is consistently offered and does not need to be earned). In addition, the student is reinforced for going progressively longer periods without doing the self-injurious behavior.

For example, a student with intellectual disability and ASD was repetitively sucking his fingers, which caused skin abrasions. A baseline assessment indicated that he sucked his fingers approximately every five minutes. The QABF assessment indicated that the major function of this behavior was to provide "nonsocial" (e.g., automatic sensory) reinforcement. The therapist determined that the student sucked his fingers seemingly to make the fingers wet and to provide oral stimulation in the mouth. Through a preference assessment, the therapist found that "water play" and a "chocolate-flavored chewy" were the student's favorite activities that more appropriately provided matching sensory input, so they were regularly offered as non-contingent reinforcements. In addition, the student was reinforced for going six minutes without sucking his hand.

The previously mentioned **redirection**, **breaks**, **self-management**, and **tolerance for delay** strategies are all evidence-based behavioral strategies. The **conditioned calm recall** and **sensory matching** strategies are based on behavioral principles but have been adapted to meet the needs of students with complex behavioral challenges such as combined intellectual, developmental, and sensory modulation challenges as well as post-traumatic stress disorder. The **conditioned calm recall** and **sensory matching** strategies are consistent with positive behavioral support but have been extended through the use of clinical reasoning. Integrating the behavioral and sensory modulation approaches can be extremely helpful for students with complex behavioral challenges.[14]

Pre-correction involves proactively attempting to avoid behavioral problems that have occurred in the past by changing the antecedents in order to increase the student's success. For example, if a student has difficulties during an assembly, the teacher can use a variety of pre-corrections before the next assembly. Pre-corrections could include making a list of assembly rules for the class, offering rewards for appropriate behavior during the assembly, providing noise-canceling headphones to students before the assembly, and increasing teacher supervision. Another important classroom-wide application of pre-correction involves the evidence-based teaching and review of a few consistent expectations, such as respectfulness and routines ("one person speaking speaks until they are finished").[15]

FAB FUNCTIONALLY ALERT BEHAVIOR STRATEGIES

Practice saying is useful for students who have difficulty appropriately asking for help when they are upset. At a time when the student is calm, they repeatedly practice a statement that is appropriate for use when asking for assistance. For example, a student who had tactile defensiveness swore and screamed after feeling a tag that his mother had forgotten to remove from his shirt. When nothing was bothering him he practiced repeatedly saying, "Please cut off the tag." The student was assisted and rewarded for asking for help in this appropriate manner.

The **Coping card**, **FAB Turtle**, *3-Comic*, *Character comic*, *Praxis comic*, and *Rainbow goal* are unique adaptations of popular clinical intervention strategies to help enable students with complex behavioral challenges to plan, describe, and use visual supports to organize their goals and actions.

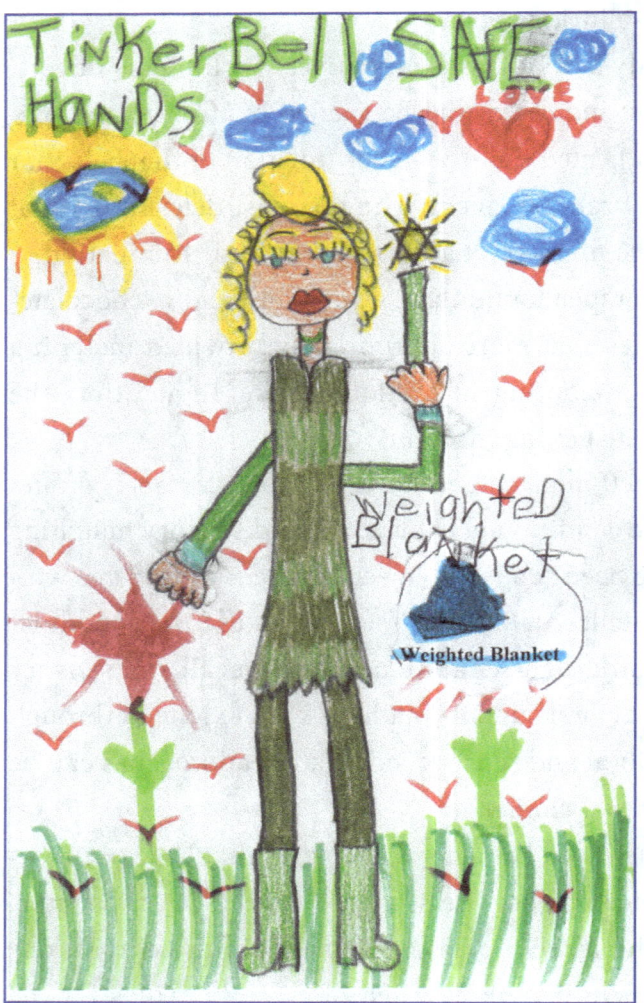

The **Coping card** is an original FAB Strategies intervention that concisely integrates the child's preferred interest, behavioral goal (e.g., a positive action that is the opposite of their inappropriate behavior), coping strategies, adaptive equipment, and reinforcement schedule on a laminated index card. For example, a student who frequently bit her hand when peers teased her helped construct a coping card.

The student first draws or places a sticker of their preferred interest—in this case, Tinker Bell—in the center of the Coping card, then writes their behavioral goal above it. Goals are developed that are the positive opposite of their problematic behavior (e.g., safe hands depicting no biting). The student colors, cuts out, and pastes their most effective coping strategy for helping with goal attainment (e.g., weighted blanket use, taken from the FAB Trigger & Coping forms). On the reverse side of the Coping card is the student's reinforcement plan: "Safe hands (e.g., not biting myself) for ten consecutive minutes earns one sticker (five stickers = one toy)." The **Coping card** is worn or posted on the desk to remind the student and all staff members of the behavioral goal, preferred interest, coping strategy, and reinforcement schedule.

The **FAB turtle** strategy is an adaptation of the PATHS turtle technique for preschoolers (www.challengingbehavior.org). The **FAB turtle** adapts the PATHS turtle technique for students with

POSITIVE BEHAVIOR SUPPORT STRATEGIES

special needs. The procedure is as follows:[16] 1) Stop immediately after noticing your environmental and body triggers. 2) Go to the classroom sensory coping area. 3) Do your individualized coping strategies in the sensory coping area. 4) When you are sure you will not act aggressively, return to your seat. 5) Later the teacher will guide you in problem solving and reward you for doing the turtle strategy to avoid aggression.

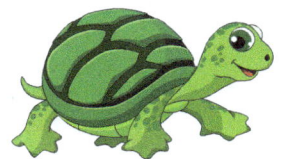

FAB Turtle Strategy

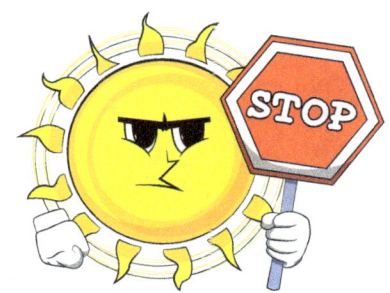

1. **NOTICE Environmental & Body Triggers STOP!!!**
2. **Go to the sensory coping area.**
3. **Do YOUR individual coping strategy.**
4. **Later, problem-solve with help.**

Domitrovich et al., 2013
Adapted with permission from Dr. Mark Greenberg
Copyright © 2019 by John Pagano, Ph.D., OTR/L, www.fabstrategies.org
Permission granted for direct use with clients.

Dialectical Behavior Therapy Strategies

Dialectical behavioral therapy includes the behavioral chain analysis strategy of assisting students in reviewing the antecedent and consequences of a specific problematic behavior so they can better understand the triggers and negative results of their actions.[16] The *3 Comic strategy* enables therapists and teachers to help students understand the triggers and problematic results of problematic behavior by drawing a three-part comic strip depicting what happened before and after their problematic target behavior. Three comics are constructed using drawings and captions. The child begins by drawing comic 2 depicting the problematic behavior; draws comic 1 next, showing the antecedent trigger; and finally comic 3 illustrating the consequences. It can be done with the child when they are calm after the problematic behavior and can be reviewed repeatedly.

FAB FUNCTIONALLY ALERT BEHAVIOR STRATEGIES

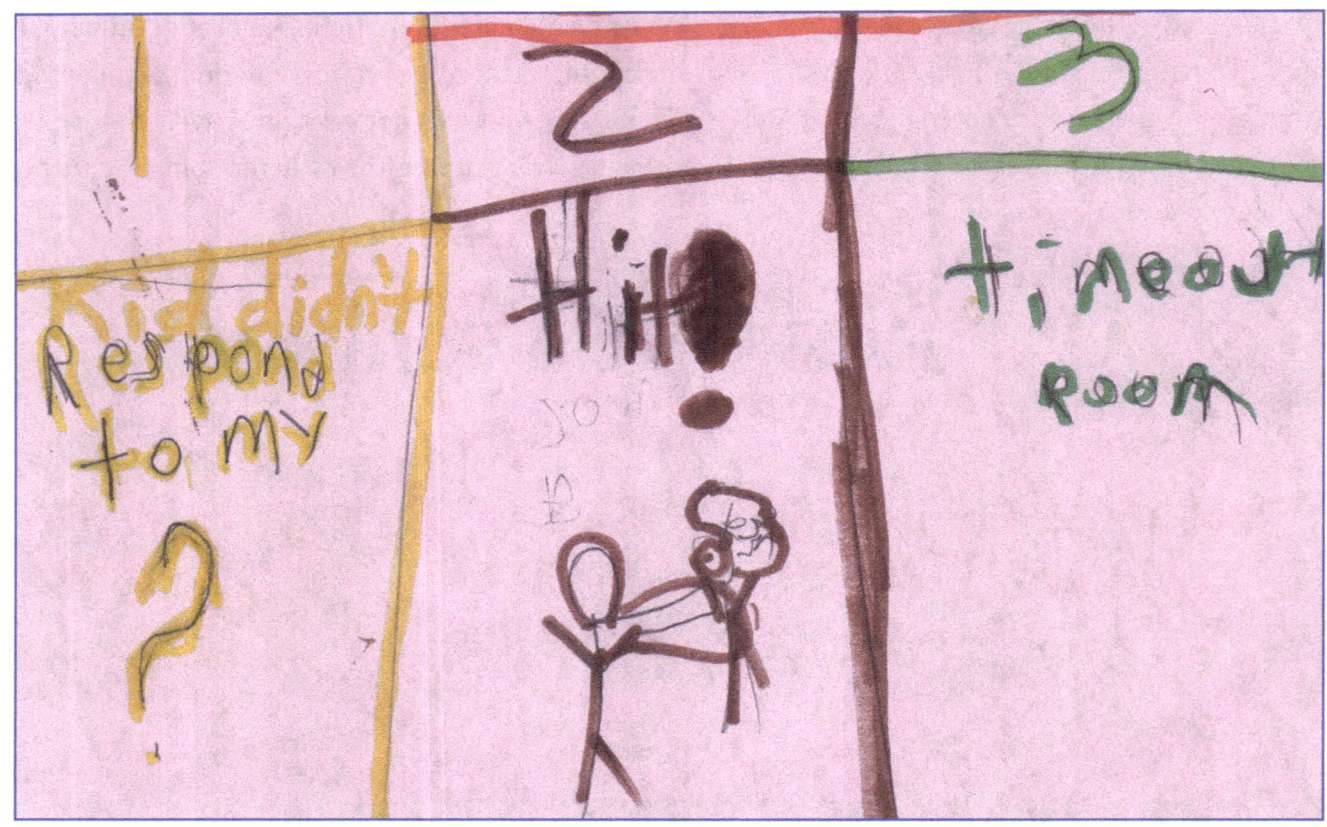

The *character comic* strategy has students develop, draw, and use a comic picture to identify a major value that motivates them toward achieving their behavior goal. Students identify a value or quality they want to convey and a superhero whom they admire who will inspire them to demonstrate this value. Superhero comics are drawn or colored with captions such as "Strong," "Assertive," "Kind," or "Hardworking."

The *praxis comic* strategy helps students understand and sequentially follow multiple-step activities. Below is the four-part FAB Praxis comic created and used by a small occupational therapy group. Group members are guided to describe, draw, and color four comics depicting the sequential components followed during each group. The students dictate and write the captions of the group sequence. The therapeutic rationale for each of the group steps is described in parentheses after the steps depicted: 1) Move the chairs (e.g., specifically involving slow, linear movement combined with deep pressure through the joints to facilitate self-regulation). 2) Throw the ball underhand (a sequential movement task that is combined with the verbal expression of feelings). 3) Sit (a calming activity during which students construct a feeling wheel or coping card, given the environmental structure of a seated position). 4) Play Frisbee, ending the group (e.g., the final routine regularly carried out before transitioning from the group by moving the chairs back to their original position and resuming class participation).

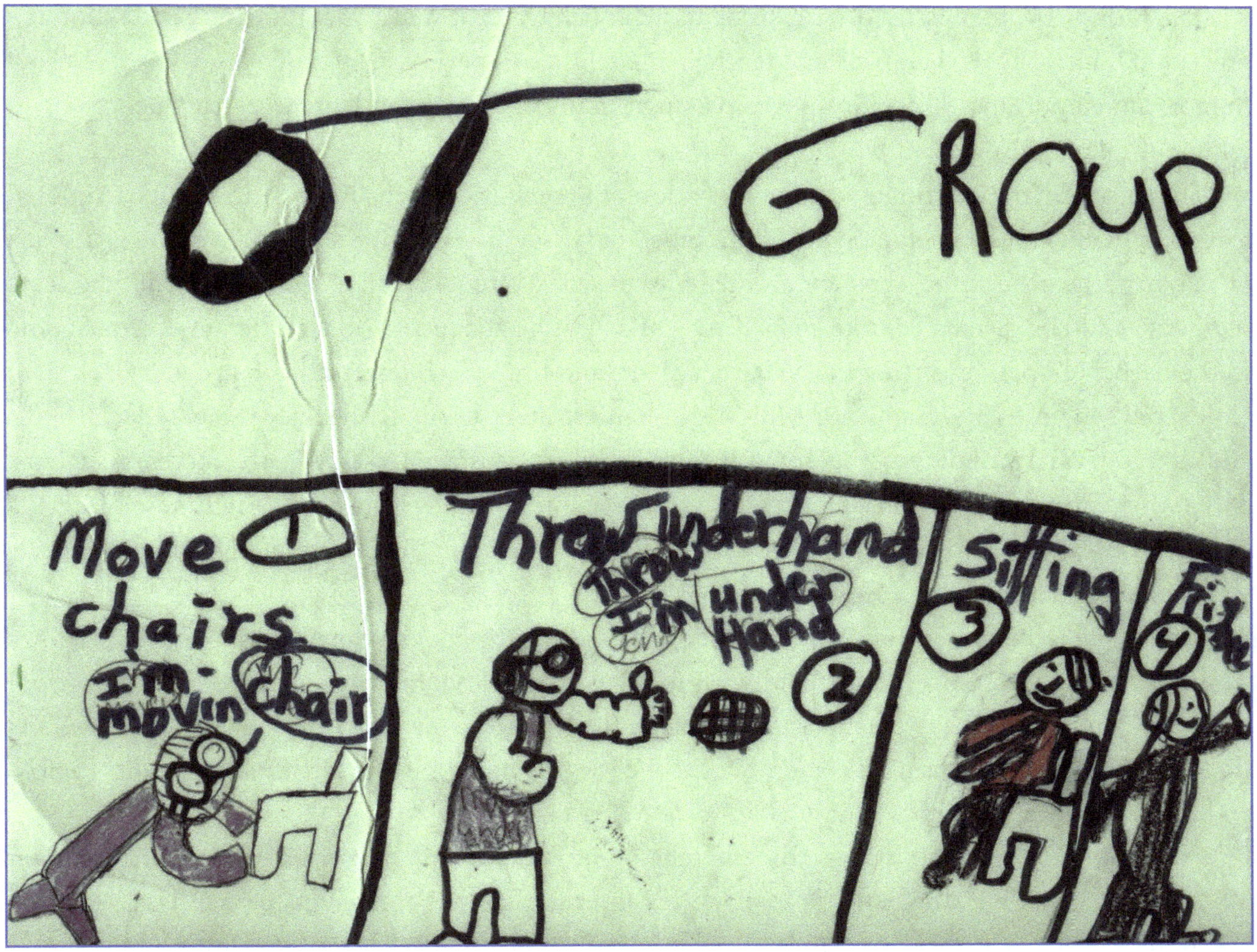

POSITIVE BEHAVIOR SUPPORT STRATEGIES

Praxis comic depicting procedures for an occupational therapy small group

Rainbow goal is an art activity that guides students in developing a behavioral goal related to their values and identifying the reinforcer that most effectively helps them attain their goal.

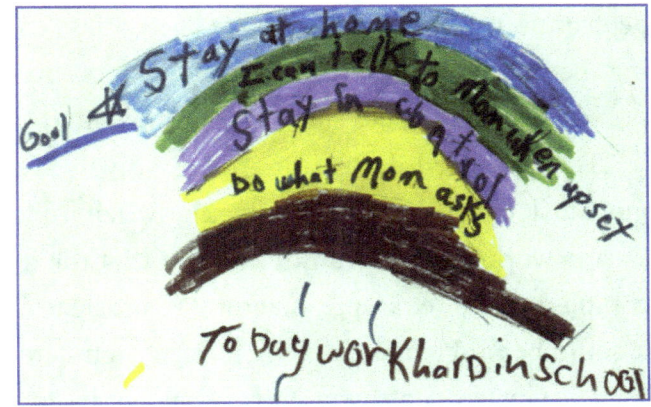

The students begin by drawing a star or pot of gold, which represents their most important goal. Next, they draw four separately colored rainbow bands beneath the star or pot of gold; these represent the steps needed—the specific things they need to do (rather than what they need to avoid doing)—to achieve their goal. The final rainbow is what they need to do immediately and is paired with a sticker system or tangible reinforcers.

FAB FUNCTIONALLY ALERT BEHAVIOR STRATEGIES

The **humor** strategy is used with students who behave best when prompts and redirection are presented humorously. Therapists and teachers model the ask permission to kid strategy before using humor. It is important to specifically avoid using this strategy with students who react negatively to joking or take kidding literally.

The **desensitization** strategy is an adaptation of systematic desensitization to reduce irrational fears in students with developmental and intellectual disabilities. While students are eating a snack or playing a favorite game, they are gradually exposed to situations they fear. A student who fears haircuts would be given a favorite snack first while looking at a picture of a barber, next while going to the barber shop, then sitting in the barber chair, and finally, while getting a haircut.

Partial sentences are a motivating fill-in-the-blank strategy to simultaneously promote social skills and literacy. **Partial sentences** begin with topics that are most motivating to the student, such as, "My favorite team is . . ." The sentences progress to express feelings, such as, "Right now I feel . . ." Finally, the teacher can facilitate social skills with this example: "There are many things I can say when I meet a new student. Here is my list: _____."

Scaffolding writing uses drawing and writing to assist young and developmentally delayed students simultaneously both with literacy and with following the *play plan-review* strategy for improved behavior. For example, the teacher can use *scaffolding writing* to assist a preschool student who is throwing blocks in the learning center. The teacher begins by asking the girl what she wants to play, and the student says, "I am Mommy."

The therapist or teacher draws three blanks on an index card and writes beneath them, "I am Mommy." The student draws pictures or writes in each blank to represent the words. Using this scaffolding writing, the teacher brings the student to the pretend-play area, helps her find the dress-up corner (e.g., redirecting her from throwing blocks), plays dress-up like Mommy with her, then reviews with the girl the activities they did together.

Preferred tasks involve selecting activities that motivate students and match their preferences, interests, and developmental level and chronological age. A preference assessment can be done to determine students' most preferred activities. Therapists and teachers are particularly skilled at finding the individualized developmentally appropriate activities that students enjoy doing. The students' preferred tasks are best for teaching them and promoting appropriate behavior.

The **preferred distractor** strategy involves selecting an item the student likes in order to promote task completion. It is particularly helpful for reducing inappropriate behaviors that are used to escape work. It's important to ensure that the item used as a distractor does not interfere with task completion. For example, listening to music is a good distractor for facilitating seated attention, but it could be problematic during math assignments because it interferes with attention to the teacher.

The **choices** strategy improves behavior by consistently offering empowering choices in a calm, non-threatening manner. The number and type of choices provided depend on the student's developmental level. Experienced therapists and teachers can consistently provide choices without compromising their behavior goals. For example, "Do you want to use a blue pen or a black pen?" "Do you want to come now or in a minute?" "Do you want to walk next to me or have me hold your hand?"

Functional Communication Strategies

Functional communication training offers occupational, speech/language, and mental health therapists the opportunity to eliminate negative behavior (e.g., to get attention, to obtain tangible objects, or to escape demands) by teaching the student an appropriate way to get their needs met.[17] This can be done through the use of visual if-then pictures (as described in Chapter 1) and by teaching the student to use the mand or break mand to appropriately communicate their needs or escape demands. The **mand** strategy involves teaching a method of communication to replace aggressive or other inappropriate behavior.[18]

A **mand** can use sign language or verbal words or phrases to appropriately obtain sensory activities and other reinforcement and to get a break from demands. Students with developmental disabilities may initially overuse the break signal to get out of tasks, but it is important to always immediately respect this request if it significantly reduces aggression. The next step is to reduce demand levels by two-thirds, but only reinforce the student if the task is accomplished.

For example, a student I worked with who had autism spectrum disorder was prompted to color within the lines. Usually he was able to complete this task, but on occasion he had difficulty, became frustrated, and hit the teacher. In conjunction with the teacher and speech/language pathologist, I taught the student to say "No thank you" as a **break mand**. All staff members began letting the student immediately escape an activity after he said, "No thank you." Use of the **break mand** eliminated aggression against staff. As expected, however, a new problem developed: Whenever we asked him to color, the student stated, "No thank you." Thus the requirement for getting reinforcement was reduced by two-thirds; instead of needing to color within the lines to receive rewards, he was rewarded for scribbling and any attempts to color. Expectations were gradually increased from this simpler level.[19]

The **intersperse learned tasks** strategy improves motivation in students with frustration tolerance challenges by alternating learned problems with new challenges, so the learned tasks are reinforced while new challenges are being introduced. **Intersperse learned tasks** is particularly useful for students with high intelligence and low self-control. Instead of giving a student ten new math problems, the teacher would intersperse five new math problems that teach all of those concepts among five math problems the student has already mastered. **Intersperse learned tasks** can also be used to intersperse mastered homework problems with challenging problems, thereby reducing homework time and thus frustration.[18]

FAB FUNCTIONALLY ALERT BEHAVIOR STRATEGIES

Priming involves previewing a new environment, people, and materials before they need to be used or interacted with. Research shows that priming improves behavior and learning in students with autism spectrum and other developmental disorders. For example, a student entering kindergarten in two weeks would visit his classroom and his teacher, and be given his books, before the start of the school year. It is most effective to use the actual items involved in a particular program and for the preview to be situated near the time the program will begin.

Prompts are given based on students' developmental needs, giving them the least amount of assistance required to maintain socially appropriate behavior. Teachers or therapists who used developmentally appropriate engaging activities, curriculum modifications, and least-to-most prompting found significantly reduced aggression in students with intellectual disabilities and autism spectrum disorder.[19] The ultimate goal is for students to independently use cognitive prompts to behave appropriately. An example of *cognitive prompts* is a typical second-grade student who remembers that they are expected to walk in class and follow this direction.

Verbal prompts involve teachers or therapists providing verbal assistance with appropriate behavior, such as when a kindergarten teacher says "Walk" to a student who is running. *Visual prompts* involve using gestures or pictures, such as gesturing to stop to a student who is running or holding up a stop sign with the word "Walk" printed on it. Some students respond best only to visual prompts, whereas others behave better if teachers simultaneously gesture and say, "Walk."

Physical prompts include hands-on physical assistance that can vary as needed from minimal (up to one-quarter of the effort involved in the task) to maximal (more than three-quarters of the effort involved). An example of a physical prompt is the teacher taking the hand of a student who is running and encouraging the child to walk along with her. The student can then be reinforced for this behavior.

Reinforce attempts is an evidence-based strategy from pivotal response training (PRT) that reinforces students for demonstrating significant effort even if the student does not answer correctly. PRT reinforces good effort in order to developmentally promote motivation. This is a useful strategy for many students and teaches them to work hard. For example, if a student shows extensive effort in solving a math problem, he is still given a sticker even though he must also be told that the answer is incorrect. This strategy is used for encouraging the developmentally important skills of motivation and good effort.

The **reinforce appropriate** strategy is an evidence-based intervention that is sometimes jokingly referred to as "being caught being good." Although universally accepted as effective, it is difficult to do, particularly in a group or classroom in which many students have complex behavioral challenges. Consider a student who frequently yells out the answer rather than raising their hand. Immediately after this student raises their hand and waits to be called on, the teacher specifically praises this behavior. The teacher might say, "Excellent job showing respect by raising your hand and waiting to be called on before giving the correct answer."[14]

POSITIVE BEHAVIOR SUPPORT STRATEGIES

A **point chart**, sometimes also referred to as a sticker chart, is a useful strategy for students above a five-year developmental level. Points are awarded for behavior that is the positive opposite of their inappropriate behavior. The most problematic negative behavior is addressed first. For example, a student who hits peers on average half the time during transitions is awarded ten points for keeping safe hands with peers during transitions. He is awarded two points for practicing to keep safe hands during transitions and ten points whenever he indeed does keep safe hands during transitions. The student can cash in his points for varied levels of reward.[20]

Tangible reinforcement occurs when teachers or therapists give specific items (e.g., favorite food or toys) immediately after a student performs a desired behavior. Although some schools dislike this strategy, it can be particularly effective for young students and those with significant developmental disabilities. It is important that the student be unable to obtain this tangible reinforcement from anyone without earning it, or its value will be reduced. For students with severe developmental disabilities, therapists often are particularly skilled at determining the tangible reinforcement because of their knowledge of the student's sensory needs and developmental level.

CHAPTER

PHYSICAL SELF-REGULATION STRATEGIES

The physical self-regulation strategies are developmentally sequenced activities that can be embedded in the daily routine to improve a student's behavioral functioning. Here, these activities are presented in a developmental sequence that makes them easier to use with students of various ages and developmental levels. The physical self-regulation activities include clinically proven ways to modulate arousal level and active, multisensory learning opportunities. These strategies involve sequential bimanual activities that can be used in conjunction with verbal strategies to promote a student's awareness of the relationship between their arousal level, feelings, and behavior.[1]

Fitness Strategies

The **push wall** strategy asks students to press forcefully on a wall for ten seconds while standing with both elbows bent slightly and hands open. **Push wall** is an isometric contraction exercise that provides calming, deep-pressure input through the arms to modulate arousal. Students can do this exercise individually or with the entire class. **Push wall** can be embedded in the daily routine for self-regulation.

Push wall is a fun movement break that is particularly useful with preschool and early elementary school classes (e.g., the teacher says she needs the class to push on the wall to make her room larger, but warns them that this may anger the teacher next door, whose room will shrink). It is helpful to have students count out loud to ensure that they do not hold their breath. Once it is learned, push wall can be done independently to regulate arousal. *Push desk* is a similar activity that is even easier to embed in a student's daily routine as a coping strategy. It involves pressing down forcefully on a desktop for ten seconds.

In t*all kneeling push hands*, the student faces the teacher and presses on his hands to move the teacher from a tall kneeling to a knee sitting position. In this way the student receives touch in a nonthreatening manner, and the amount of deep pressure can be graded through the teacher's level

■ 65 ■

of resistance. In *tall kneeling push therapy ball*, the student and teacher face each other at a distance of eight feet and roll the therapy ball back and forth.

The *tall kneeling push hands* strategy introduces interpersonal touch and deep-pressure input during a nonthreatening, playful activity. The therapist and client are both in the tall kneeling position, and the client—keeping the trunk stable so they do not fall down onto the mat, thereby losing a point—pushes the therapist back ten times, earning a point each time. This strategy provides linear vestibular movement and deep-pressure proprioceptive resistance, which facilitate sensory modulation and self-regulation in most clients. The therapist grades his resistance to match the strengthening, dynamic balance, and proprioceptive needs of the client.

Tall kneeling push hands is particularly helpful for clients who have a history of physical or sexual abuse, because it empowers them to push the therapist away and provides interpersonal touch, but in a playful manner. The therapist can joke that if he removes his hands quickly and the client falls to the mat, a pretend alligator will eat the client's fingernails, and a point toward the ten pushes is deducted, requiring them to do extra work. The therapist can also tumble backward in a playful, exaggerated manner. *Tall kneeling push therapy ball* provides the same sensory input; but through pushing a therapy ball back and forth, it avoids the need for interpersonal touch.

Push-ups are an excellent sensory coping strategy for students who enjoy doing them, because they can be done independently to modulate arousal by both sensory under-responsive students and sensory over-responsive students. Simultaneously receiving deep pressure through the joints and performing slow, linear movement is a common component of many of the physical self-regulation activities that seem to promote self-regulation. Because push-ups are such a popular exercise, they are particularly useful in a classroom and as a coping strategy for mainstreamed students with behavioral challenges.

Several alternatives, from easiest to most difficult, are offered here for grading push-ups to match students' individual deep-pressure needs, strength, and gross motor development. The simplest is **wall push-ups**, which the student does while standing with their hands against a wall. The difficulty can be incrementally increased by doing *marine wall push-ups*, with an adult leaning on the student as they do push-ups against the wall and clap between each repetition. The last, and most difficult, are regular *push-ups*, which can be made more difficult by increasing the repetitions.

The usefulness of **push-ups** in the mainstream environment became clear to me when I decided to better integrate occupational therapy (OT) into the school culture. A student in middle school refused to participate in OT with me because "Therapy is only for the retarded kids. I don't need it." This statement angered me, so I asked my son, who was also in middle school at the time, what I needed to do to be part of the school like the teachers are. He said, "Dad, you need a bulletin board." I got permission to make an OT bulletin board, then asked my son how I could have the best bulletin board in the school. He said, "You need to involve the popular kids." Although I was initially skeptical,

PHYSICAL SELF-REGULATION STRATEGIES

all the middle-school students I questioned named the same three students, so I found them and got their permission to let me trace their hands and use their first names on my bulletin board. I made a wall push-ups OT bulletin board that became extremely popular. As students walked through the halls they stopped to do wall-push-ups in the handprints of the popular students.

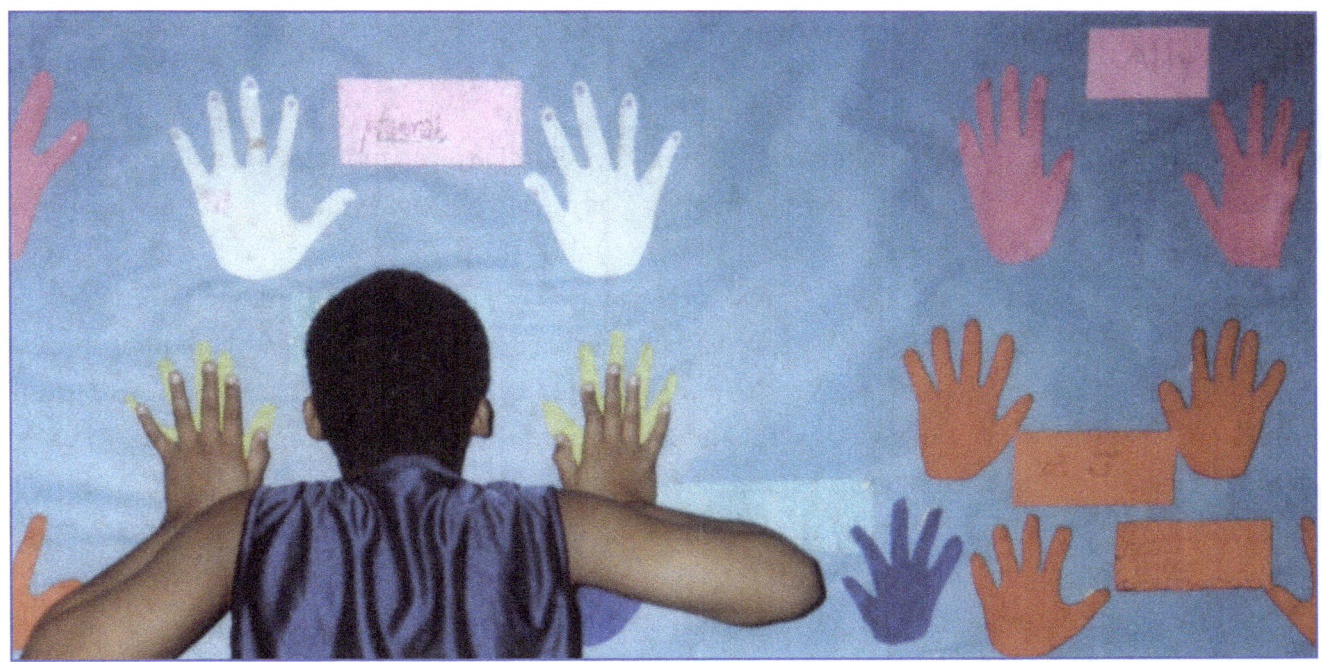

Once a student can easily do regular push-ups, the difficulty can be increased by having them use a bar to do *pull-ups*. *Pull-ups* provide pressure input through the arms while still providing linear movement and can have the added benefit of providing input through arm traction when the student is initially hanging from the bar. When students are doing pull-ups, it is important to ensure that they maintain appropriate form to receive maximal benefit from the exercise.

Exercise band activities use either a TheraBand or exercise tubing (for students who prefer greater sensory input). The resistance of TheraBands and exercise tubing is graded by color: Darker colors (e.g., red) indicate greater resistance, and lighter colors (e.g., yellow) indicate progressively less resistance. The therapist or teacher can provide even less resistance by giving more slack and using longer bands. The first and most basic activity involves bringing the band forward ten times to punch the adult's hand. The second movement involves bringing the arm straight down, extending the elbow. The third and most complex activity is pulling the band in to cross the midline. The latter is a complex task for many students and is thought to promote the brain hemisphere coordination required for many academic skills such as simultaneously holding a piece of paper and writing.

Cardio machines can be extremely useful for adolescents who have aggressive behavior, as long as they are carefully supervised. **Cardio machines** tend to be popular with teens, providing cardiovascular exercise that reduces stress, promotes physical health, helps reduce depression, and promotes

FAB FUNCTIONALLY ALERT BEHAVIOR STRATEGIES

neurological resiliency. Cardio machines, along with other equipment, are usually found in fitness rooms and can be used if students adhere to the clothing and safety rules of the fitness room.

Walking, *biking*, *riding a scooter*, *swimming*, *basketball*, *soccer*, and *dance* are alternative strategies that provide linear vestibular and proprioceptive deep-pressure input through the joints to promote body awareness. It is important to discover activities such as these that the student likes and that can be integrated into their home routine.

The **weight lift** strategy is popular among many teenagers and can promote body awareness through intense proprioceptive input. Weightlifting is a helpful arousal modulation activity for many older adolescents, providing deep-pressure input for body awareness and calming through the use of a socially acceptable strengthening exercise. While weightlifting, students need to be closely monitored to avoid overexertion and injury, but a universal gym offers a relatively safe option.

Similar to weightlifting, the **punch heavy bag** strategy can provide deep pressure for body awareness, and it enables students to express their anger without hurting themselves or others. I often introduce the punch heavy bag activity to students who injure their hands by punching walls or self-injure because they are unable to express their anger. While this strategy is often controversial, as it provides students with boxing gloves and lets them hit a heavy bag, it is safe to use when adults are supervising the activity. If students visualize hurting others or if they ever become aggressive after this activity, the therapist or teacher needs to immediately discontinue its use. However, punch heavy bag also offers an opportunity to discuss how feelings of anger differ from, but can be related to, aggressive behavior.

As with the increasingly challenging activities that follow it, **prone on therapy ball: hands rock** independently provides students with simultaneous linear movement and pressure through their arm joints to facilitate self-regulation. The student begins by kneeling in front of a therapy ball. Next, the student rolls their stomach and trunk over the therapy ball, placing both of their open hands on the floor. Finally, pushing themselves backwards with both hands, the student returns to a kneeling position in front of the therapy ball. This sequence is repeated ten times. **Prone on therapy ball: wheelbarrow walk** incrementally increases the difficulty while helping with self-calming. The student pushes themselves onto their hands, wheelbarrow walks forward as far as possible, then wheelbarrow walks back to the starting position ten times. For younger students, this can be done as a game with the parent, teacher, or therapist holding the student's legs.

Mini-trampoline jumping provides cardio exercise as well as simultaneous deep pressure and linear movement sensory input. However, **mini-trampoline jumping** should be monitored so the student doesn't become overly aroused and as a consequence behave inappropriately. It may be helpful to slow the jumping speed (e.g., clap a rhythm to guide the student in jumping at a slower speed). Another helpful strategy to modulate the vestibular input of jumping on a mini-trampoline is for the therapist or teacher to add more deep pressure by holding the student's hands or providing pressure downward on both of the student's shoulders ("dribbling" the student like a basketball).

The **play structure strategy** is useful for occupational, physical, speech/language, mental health, and behavioral therapists, as well as for teachers and administrators, to help students learn to use the playground without being aggressive (e.g., pushing other children down). During individual therapy sessions, the therapist gives the student an opportunity to select one limited area of the playground where they will increase structure (e.g., around the sliding board, using a jump rope to define the area). Students then play for a minimal period of time in the selected area, clean up the area, and select the next area for play. The therapist monitors these rules, providing structure and immediate consequences when the student does not follow the rules or engages in aggressive behavior (e.g., if the student pushes a peer or leaves the designated area, the student must go inside). The therapist gradually begins to monitor the student from farther away while implementing rules and environmental adaptations that enable the student to use the playground without showing aggressive behavior.

Integrating Aerobic, Coordination, and Mindfulness Exercises

Several FAB Strategies include aerobic, coordination, and mindfulness exercises specifically shown to improve preschoolers' development of executive functions including inhibitory control, working memory, and flexible thinking.[2] In general, to promote mindfulness for increased attention, it is important to proceed quickly enough that the student or group is willing to participate in the activity, but as slowly as possible so they are able to experience it. Research supports the efficacy of goal-directed yoga, horseback riding, and arousal level modulation for improving students' self-control.[3]

In addition to focusing on the body to promote body awareness and relaxation, many mindfulness, yoga, and movement activities also involve sequential movement, which promotes attention and visual-motor skills. Many movement activities either involve the same side (e.g., right arm and right leg) or cross the midline (e.g., right arm and left leg). Preliminary research suggests that same-side movement improves learning retention, whereas crossing the midline improves bilateral coordination.[4]

If done with sufficient intensity, all of the physical self-regulation strategies also have the potential to provide cardiovascular exercise, which has been shown to significantly increase elementary students' attention[5] and classroom learning.[6] Cardiovascular exercise has also been shown to significantly increase self-control in students who are obese and sedentary.[5] Research with students who have autism spectrum disorders shows that cardiovascular exercise significantly improves attention and learning,[7] and preliminary evidence suggests that movement activities improve mental health.[8]

FAB FUNCTIONALLY ALERT BEHAVIOR STRATEGIES

The *back rolls* strategy provides linear vestibular movement with deep proprioceptive pressure. *Back rolls* begin with students sitting on a mat. Then they simply roll backward until the neck touches the ground, then return to sitting, repeating the motion. Therapists can linearly rock children with physical challenges by embracing the child in their lap while doing the movement. *Child's pose* is done by bending the knees so they are moved on the calves while stretching both arms forward bringing the forehead to the floor.

Research suggests that learning new sequential bimanual tasks may facilitate myelination in the corpus callosum and communication between brain hemispheres, which allows right hemisphere feelings, such as rage and fear, to be modulated by language reference ("I feel hungry, tired, and angry") in the left hemisphere. In addition, sequential bimanual movements require students to concentrate in order to promote a state of mindfulness that can decrease stress. The **flex & extend shoulder & ankle** strategy provides developmentally graded mindfulness activities, presented in increasingly complex developmental order; these help to decrease stress.[4]

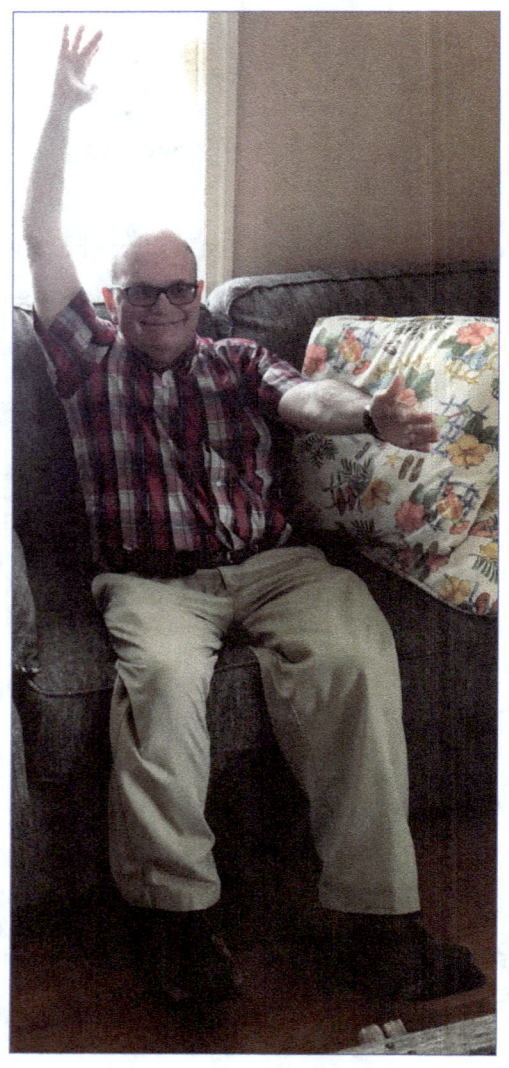

From a developmental perspective, the most basic of these strategies is **flex & extend shoulder & ankle same side** (e.g., simultaneously flexing the left shoulder and ankle). Next in developmental complexity is **flex & extend shoulder and ankle opposite sides** (e.g., simultaneously flexing the left shoulder and right ankle). The most developmentally complex is **flex & extend shoulder & ankle opposite, adding same shoulder halfway up & down**, in which a student flexes and extends the shoulder and ankle on opposite sides while moving the opposite arm to accompany the arm movement initially halfway up the body then remaining still before accompanying it the final halfway down (e.g., simultaneously flexing the left shoulder and right ankle, raising the right shoulder halfway up initially then the final halfway down accompanying the left shoulder). Students can do the **flex & extend shoulder & ankle** strategies while seated or when lying on their back on a mat.

A developmental sequence of progressively more challenging hand-to-knee activities promotes bilateral coordination and midline crossing. The simplest task is to have students use **both hands**, with the fingers interlaced, and bring each knee up to touch their palms, alternating knees. Once students can do this, they can be asked to do **hand**

PHYSICAL SELF-REGULATION STRATEGIES

same-side knee (e.g., bringing the right hand to their right knee then their left hand to their left knee, alternating back and forth). The next task is **hand opposite knee** (e.g., bringing the right hand to the left knee and the left hand to the right knee). The next, progressively more difficult task is **Same-side knee-*Eyes down right*** (e.g., sequentially bringing the hands to the knee on the same side while focusing both eyes down diagonally to the right). Finally, students are asked to do **Opposite knee-*Eyes up left*** (e.g., sequentially bringing their hands to the knee on the opposite side while focusing both eyes diagonally up to the left).

A developmental sequence of progressively more challenging unilateral and bilateral movements can be done to improve bilateral coordination and midline-crossing skills. The first movement in the sequence is "air draw" a diagonal with the index finger to repeatedly form a **diagonal**, moving the finger in the air from the top left to the bottom right. The next action is to repeatedly "air draw" a diagonal from the top right to the bottom left.

Continuing the developmental progression, the therapist leads students in air drawing a large "**X**" repeatedly across the center of their body. Finally, students do an **infinity I** by repeatedly air drawing an infinity sign with one hand across the center of their body.

The next developmental progression is to sequentially use both hands, moving from the outside to the center, so together they form the **alternate I** infinity sign. After the students are able to do the **alternate I**, they progress to **I visually track**, where they air draw the infinity sign but also follow its movement with their eyes.

The next developmental task is the **Elbow I**. First, students do a **pre-check twist** by putting both hands on their hips and noticing how far and easily they can twist to each side. Students then use each elbow to repetitively "air draw" infinity signs, proceeding as far back to as far forward as possible with each elbow. After this, students do a post-check by again placing their hands on their hips and noticing whether they can twist any farther or more easily than they did at pre-check.

The final developmental task is **symmetry**, involving mirror-image drawing with both hands (e.g., making a heart shape). Symmetry can be done with both hands drawing in the air, drawing in shaving cream, or holding flashlights. Also, symmetry is fun when students can use a different color markers or sponge paint in each hand to draw.[8]

Visual-Motor and Movement FAB Strategies

Wall ball is a two-person visual-motor and motor planning game in which one partner throws the ball underhand to an opponent. If the opponent catches the ball before it bounces, he gets two points; catching it after one bounce earns a point; and letting it bounce twice or missing it results in zero points. The first player to get thirty points wins. With extremely competitive students, the game

FAB FUNCTIONALLY ALERT BEHAVIOR STRATEGIES

works best cooperatively, with both partners helping each other reach a joint total of thirty points as quickly as possible.

Using strong kinesthetic skills to improve visual perception for functional writing, **letter ball** helps students at or above a second-grade academic level practice letter formation. The therapist says a letter and the student tries to "print" it on the wall by drawing the shape of the letter with the ball. The movement of the ball to form the letter "d," for example, seems to be helpful for students with good kinesthetic skills who have visual perception difficulties that cause them to reverse letters. Following a sequence from least to most difficult, the student can practice drawing the letters they most commonly reverse. By proceeding developmentally, the student can practice increasingly complex lowercase letters that they usually reverse. When addressing reversals, the most common developmental progression is n, u, w, m, z, s, b, d, p, q.

Wall ball lets students with writing difficulties practice forming letters through the use of a game that does not require them to formally print. If the student "writes" the letter correctly, the therapist praises them, takes the ball, and throws it to the student, who runs for the pass. The student earns one point for each catch until ten points are scored. If the student does not form the letter correctly, the student practices forming the letter ten times with her eyes closed, with the adult guiding her hands or the ball to help the student feel how the letter is formed, if needed. Then the student forms the letter accurately with her eyes open and resumes the game.

Quadruped pass involves the student and adult each in a hands-and-knees position. Facing each other, they pass the ball back and forth cooperatively twenty to fifty times. The adult coaches the student to roll the ball by alternating hands, with the elbows partially extended and hands open. This activity provides weight bearing for proprioceptive input through the arms, weight shifting, and visual-motor coordination.

Shoot to target ball involves various size balls and baskets positioned at gradually more challenging angles and distances. This activity helps students to practice visual-motor skills. It is important to stress that this is a fun, made-up game that is never on college exams so that students can practice their skills while relaxing and having fun. **Bat ball** involves hitting a punch balloon in various and alternating ways to increase body awareness and sensory discrimination skills. Increasingly complex body parts can be chosen for use in passing the punch balloon: hand, foot, head, knee, elbow, wrist, ankle, nose, ears. Concepts of "left" and "right" arm or leg are added after the student shows awareness of the body part (e.g., hand) and are at or above a second-grade level.

Ball bounce activities involve a developmental progression of activities that bounce racquet balls.[9] The **ball bounce activities** are presented with the direction that this is silly, unimportant game, and that the goal of the game is to have fun and be nice to classmates. The ball bounce activities involve sequential bimanual activities that are fun and teach frustration tolerance.

PHYSICAL SELF-REGULATION STRATEGIES

Beanbag pass activities are a movement planning game that can be done to teach new sequential bilateral skills to encourage interactions between the brain hemispheres. The **Beanbag pass activity** begins by asking students to throw a beanbag underhand to another student, and to pass the bean bag to that same student every time. As the game progresses, the therapist can increase the complexity by adding more beanbags. Another variation of beanbag pass asks students to describe their favorite thing before throwing the beanbag. For example, the therapist poses a question (e.g., "What is your favorite color/song/coping strategy?"), and each student describes their favorite. A more developmentally complex question would ask how the students are feeling, what their criteria are when choosing a friend, or which situations cause them to become angry. The most complex question is to have the group create "I messages"; for example, "When people do _____ [e.g., call me names] I feel _____ [e.g., mad], so I would like them to _____ [e.g., please speak respectfully to me]." Students can also state positive I messages (e.g., "When people say hello to me, I feel cared about, so please say hello when you see me").

A *balance beam* or *tilt board* can improve balance and body awareness by providing students with increasingly complex opportunities to actively challenge their balance. Balance activities can also help promote students' basic body awareness (e.g., provide basic sensory awareness of the front and back surfaces as well as the top and bottom of their body). Balance reactions are introduced in a developmental sequence, with students initially improving balance forward and back. Next, use of a mini-trampoline or going under and over obstacles provides awareness of the top and bottom of the body. When providing sideways balance, the concepts "left" and "right" are introduced when the child is at or above a second-grade level.

Some students may function better after performing specific sensory strategies that prepare them for, or help them transition between, academic tasks. Some students are under-responsive to sensory input and demonstrate improved self-control and learning immediately after opportunities to jump or fall into a foam **crash pad**. It is important to ensure that the crash pad is used safely and results in improved behavior and learning after use. Under-responsive students must also be guided to ask the question, "Is that safe?" before doing crash pad activities.

Scooter board use by students under the supervision of a therapist can provide independent linear movement with deep-pressure experiences to enhance self-control. **Scooter board pull** gives active traction as input as students pull hand over hand on a rope or hold onto a scooter board and are pulled by the therapist. **Scooter board push** provides deep-pressure input as students propel the scooter board with their hands while lying on their stomach on the board. With supervision, students can also push up or down a ramp. Students can receive enhanced deep-pressure input by crashing the scooter board into cardboard blocks.

Therapist-directed use of a **suspended swing** promotes self-control and learning in some students. When initially determining the type of swinging that will be most helpful in promoting

FAB FUNCTIONALLY ALERT BEHAVIOR STRATEGIES

self-regulation, therapists should use a developmental progression. Initially, and especially when students appear to be hyper-reactive, linear **forward-back** swinging with the therapist providing firm pressure while pushing the student usually appears most clinically helpful in calming the student. Slow, linear swinging with deep-pressure pushes from the therapist can be extremely helpful for calming students when they are beginning to become upset, and doing a learning activity while swinging can help promote learning when the student begins to become too hyper-responsive to learn.[9]

Different types of suspended swings and movements can be used to individualize swinging to the student's needs. For students with a history of developmental trauma, linear motion

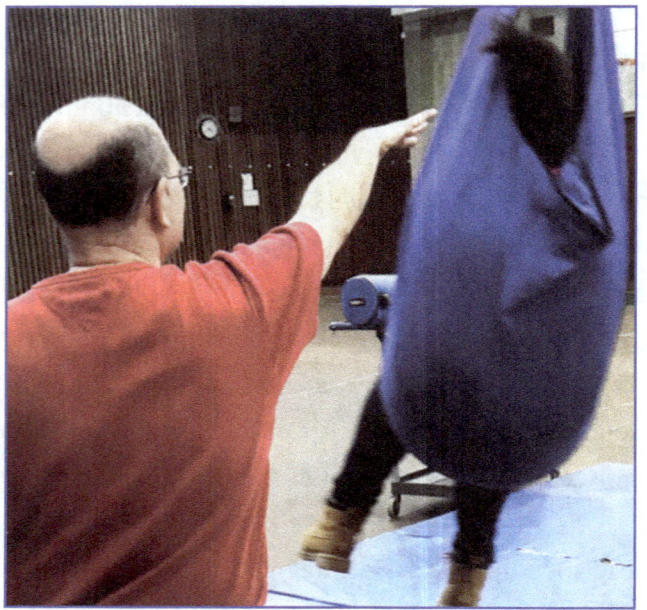

in a cuddle swing, with firm pushes from the therapist against the student's back, can facilitate calming.

After the student can tolerate forward-back swinging, and if more movement input seems to be needed, **lateral** movement can be attempted. Finally, upon request, the therapist can spin the student for brief periods to provide intense movement stimulation. The therapist should, however, carefully monitor the student's reaction during and after spinning.

Spin in a suspended swing involves carefully monitored spinning to provide increased stimulation to the vestibular system. The therapist monitors the student for changes to the autonomic nervous system (e.g., laughter, pale or red skin, sleepiness, nausea, dizziness). If negative effects are observed, the therapist must stop the spinning. With all suspended swing activities, but particularly with spinning, it is important that the therapist monitor the student's behavior for an hour after the activity, as delayed effects can be noted.

During forward-back swinging, various **throw to target** activities can be done to improve visual-motor skills. When suspension equipment is unavailable, an alternative is to use an astronaut board to provide rotary vestibular input. The crash pad, scooter board and suspended swinging strategies are only useful if done under the direction of a trained therapist. The therapist can use these strategies effectively by basing them on an individualized assessment and demonstrating that they significantly improve behavioral goal attainment.

PHYSICAL SELF-REGULATION STRATEGIES

Summary

The physical self-regulation strategies provide active sensory-motor strategies that can be embedded in the student's daily routines to improve their functional behavior. The physical self-regulation strategies are listed within individual lines of the FAB Strategies form in developmental order so that they can be easily individualized to meet the needs of students. The physical self-regulation strategies can be consistently implemented in the home, classroom, small group, and individual therapy settings.

The physical self-regulation strategies are designed to encourage collaboration between therapists, teachers, and parents. This consistency of activities and expectations across settings is extremely helpful for students with developmental and behavioral challenges. It is hoped that the FAB Strategies form can facilitate team collaboration of the physical self-regulation and other FAB Strategies areas.

Back in Chapter 1 this book presented the Environmental Adaptation strategies providing the physical structure for improved behavior. The next three chapters added sensory modulation, touch, and positive behavior support strategies that provide more advanced interventions that could meet the individual needs of students with complex behavioral challenges. This chapter presented physical self-regulation strategies, which can often be used in individual and small group intervention, as well as in classroom settings. The next chapter will describe how these various categories of FAB Strategies can be integrated into an individualized program to help students with complex behavioral challenges. Clinical examples will also be given demonstrating the use of the FAB Strategies or FAB Strategies Pre-K & Kindergarten form to develop transdisciplinary programs that are individualized for students with complex behavioral challenges.

CHAPTER 6

INDIVIDUALIZING INTERVENTION WITH THE FAB STRATEGIES FORM

Therapists and teachers can use the FAB Strategies form to guide the development of an individualized program for a student with complex behavioral challenges. As described in the introduction, all of the strategies set in boldface print in this book are included on the FAB Strategies form; the strategies set in italics can be added on the two blank lines on the bottom of the FAB Strategies form (Figure 6.1). The form is organized into four sections—environmental adaptation (section A), sensory modulation (section B), positive behavior support (section C), and physical self-regulation (section D)—to make it easier for therapists and teachers to locate and use the strategies.

One useful way therapists or teachers can initially customize the FAB Strategies form is to fill in their name and professional contact information, add at the bottom two lines of the form five to ten of their most frequently used strategies, then make copies. Before planning individualized strategies for a student, it is important that therapists develop the student's most essential behavior goal and write it at the top of the form. Given the many significant difficulties of students with complex behavioral challenges, it is important to prioritize their goals. Factors to consider when developing goals include the current classroom teacher-to-student ratio, the expected frequency and duration of therapy interventions, and the student's most likely next school setting.

The goal can be one of the goals included on the student's Individualized Education Plan (IEP), or it could be the most immediate first step toward achieving them. While developing goals, therapists and teachers should consider giving priority consideration to the following actions (from highest to least priority): physical aggression toward other students, physical aggression toward staff, self-injurious behavior, property destruction, and extremely limited attention. It is important to record baseline data regarding the frequency, duration, and extent of the targeted problematic behavior before implementing an intervention.

An important yet often neglected step before beginning treatment is to obtain a baseline of the student's current goal performance. Goals are created to develop the positive opposite of the student's most problematic behavior. For example, for a student who hits classmates, the goal may be for the student to keep safe hands toward other students for fifteen consecutive minutes. If the student currently hits other students approximately every eight minutes, the therapist or teacher would record this duration as the baseline before starting treatment. This value provides objective evidence of whether the intervention is effective. Therapists and teachers often become frustrated because, for example, after two weeks of trying an individualized program, the student is keeping safe hands with classmates for only fourteen minutes. In this case, the therapist and teacher don't realize that the student's behavior has significantly improved.

INDIVIDUALIZING INTERVENTION WITH THE FAB STRATEGIES FORM

Figure 6.1 FAB Strategies to Improve Self-Control Form

Copyright © 2019 by John Pagano, Ph.D., OTR/L, *www.fabstrategies.org*

X: therapist   √: family/teacher   A: Attachment

Client: _____ Therapist: _____ Contact: _____
Functional Goals: _____ Dates: _____

A. ENVIRONMENTAL ADAPTATION
____ Sensory coping area/Prepare-Limit-Transitions/Low noise/Headphones/Fidget-Comfort Box-Bag
____ **Ear Press/Weighted-Blanket-Pressure-Vest/Pencil grip/Chewy/Sit: Stable-Separate-Carrel-Disk**
____ Visual: List-Schedule-If then/Schedule story/Sit near teacher/Calm face/Slow: Speech-Pace
____ Choice of 1 activity from . . . 4 choices; do ____ minutes minimum; clean up before next activity

B. SENSORY MODULATION
____ Arousal level-Modulate/Coping strategies/Breathing: Hand-Bird-4462/Mindful clock: Sit-Stand
____ Freeze dance/Giant steps/Simon says/Deliver: Books-Messages-Box/Rolling to Read-Math
____ Beans & Rice-Theraputty-Sand-Playdoh-Water-Glue-Shaving cream/Self-brushing
____ Vibration/Back: X-Crawl/Tap-Press self: Fingers to ear-Head to feet/Roll therapy ball-Core
____ **Touch: Back-Arm/Head crown/Shoulders: Squeeze-Press/Spine roll/Back tech: Tap-Press**
____ **Supported sitting therapy ball: Forward & back-Up & down-Sides-Mindful clock**

C. POSITIVE BEHAVIOR SUPPORT
____ Ask permission to kid-Touch/Prompt filter speech/Invite/Will like you/Social role-play/Redirect
____ Breaks/Self-management/Tolerance for delay/Conditioned calm recall/Sensory matching
____ Pre-correction/Practice saying/Coping card/FAB Turtle/Humor/Desensitization/Partial sentences
____ Preferred: Tasks-Distractor/Choices/Break-Mand/Intersperse learned tasks/Priming/Prompts
____ Reinforce: Attempts-Appropriate-Point chart-Tangible/Desensitization/Self-management

D. PHYSICAL SELF-REGULATION
____ Push wall/Push-ups-Wall/Exercise band activities/Cardio machines/Weight lift/Punch heavy bag
____ Prone on therapy ball: Hands rock-Wheelbarrow walk/Mini-trampoline jump/Play structure
____ Flex & extend shoulder & ankle: Same-Opposite-Opposite, adding shoulder halfway up & down
____ Both-Hand: Same-side knee-*Eyes down right*/Opposite knee-*Eyes up left*
____ Diagonal-X-Infinity I-Alternate I-I visually track/Pre-check twist/Elbow I/Symmetry
____ Ball: Wall-Letter-Quadruped pass-Bat-Bounce activities/Beanbag pass activities
____ **Crash Pad/Scooter board: Pull-Push/Suspended Swing: Forward-Back-Lateral-Spin-Target**
____ Activities: _____
____ Activities: _____

www.fabstrategies.org   www.challengingbehavior.org   www.spdstar.org

References: Domitrovich et al., 2013; Koester, 2012; LaVigna & Willis, 2012; Stahmer et al., 2011

Using the FAB Strategies Form

Section A, Environmental Adaptation, begins by requiring the therapist or teacher to consider the most effective adaptive equipment and techniques to promote appropriate behavior (presented in Chapter 1). Section B, Sensory Modulation, builds on environmental adaptation strategies to help lower stress and enhance self-regulation (presented in Chapter 2). Touch strategies (presented in Chapter 3) are a component of sensory modulation strategies.

Students with developmental challenges are frequently motivated to participate in sensory modulation strategies, making them an effective means for promoting behavioral change. It is crucial for therapists and teachers to attend to the arousal level of a student with complex behavioral strategies so that the student can interact with others without being aggressive. For example, if a child rates his arousal level as "hypersensitive" after playground tasks, the therapist or teacher should assist him to calm down before he returns to class.

Section C, Positive Behavior Support, lists strategies to improve behavior and communication skills (presented in Chapter 4). Learning social and communication skills significantly improves the behavior of children with developmental and behavioral challenges. Included in this section is the bully-proof strategy to help youngsters with developmental and mental health challenges cope with verbal and physical bullying. The strategies listed in Section D, Physical Self-Regulation, promote attention, behavior, and social skills through cardiovascular, dynamic balance, sensory motor, and sequential bilateral tasks (presented in Chapter 5).

In addition to using it to help create an individualized plan to improve behavior, therapists can use the FAB Strategies form as a checklist of effective behavioral strategies; to plan an intervention before, or record an effective intervention during, sessions; to develop a transdisciplinary curriculum plan; or to use as a home or discharge program. The FAB Strategies curriculum provides practical, multidisciplinary intervention strategies that are supported by research. It gives parents, teachers, physicians, nurses, and occupational, physical, speech/language, and mental health therapists a practical guide for coordinated behavioral intervention. FAB Strategies allow for individualization, specify the goal progress and intervention methods used, and help teachers and therapists assess the efficacy of multidisciplinary interventions.

Using a student's individualized goal to guide me, I develop their treatment by checking off the line and underlining the best treatment strategies for attaining the goal. (I use a pencil so I can easily revise my notes on the form, if necessary.) It is important to select FAB Strategies that motivate the student and to embed them in the educational curriculum. I circle promising strategies that I don't have time to try now for use when I'm planning the treatment in the next intervention section. I keep each student's FAB Strategies form in a notebook and use it during evaluations and interventions.

INDIVIDUALIZING INTERVENTION WITH THE FAB STRATEGIES FORM

The most frequent application of the FAB Strategies form is to individualize and plan interventions for students with complex behavioral challenges. Therapists and teachers can fill out the FAB Strategies form for each student, with the student's goal and baseline listed at the top, and then use it during intervention and consultation sessions. During therapy and classroom consultations, therapists and teachers can use a pencil to check off the column and underline the strategies that seem to be most effective. When the therapy or consultation session concludes, therapists can circle strategies that seem promising so they can try them during the next session. The form can be filled out completely later as part of the home program, or it can be given to other professionals when the client advances to the next grade or changes therapy settings.

Therapists and teachers can eventually use the FAB Strategies form to quickly develop consistent multidisciplinary intervention programs for students with complex behavioral challenges. While schools stress inclusion and multidisciplinary intervention programs, professionals are seldom given sufficient time to work collaboratively to implement them. Students with complex behavioral challenges often become upset when various staff members use different rules, rewards, and interventions. The FAB Strategies form can be brought to IEP meetings, where it can be used to quickly develop multidisciplinary programs and ensure that students are making progress toward their goals and that all team members working with those students are consistently applying the same strategies.

The FAB Strategies form is for developing suggestions for home programs for use in other disciplines and by families. When developing programs for teachers and parents to implement, it is best for the therapist to include one or two strategies they have found consistently helpful in improving behavior. By limiting consultation suggestions, the teacher and parent are more likely to implement the strategies and seek further intervention suggestions. Also, before assigning a strategy as part of a home program, be sure that the strategy has been taught well enough to the staff or parent that they can use it effectively. I give the teacher or parent a copy of the form listing the suggested strategies, keep the original for my records and to guide further consultations, and note the date and person with whom I consulted.

A few FAB Strategies options (listed in blue) are included for use by occupational, physical, or speech/language therapists. As mentioned previously, two blank lines are shown at the bottom of the form, where strategies not listed on the form can be added. Below these lines is a list of free online resources that a therapist can underline as recommendations. At the bottom of the form is a line for the parent's or guardian's signature, which indicates that they understand and agree with the strategies used. This is a quick way to obtain parental consent for the use of adaptive equipment and strategies, and it is particularly important before implementing touch pressure strategies or using adaptive equipment such as a weighted vest.

It is important to start by listing only strategies that have been used for at least two weeks (consistent use for two weeks allows one to determine whether a strategy is effective or needs to be modified) and that are consistently helpful in improving the student's behavior. If a staff member loses their form, simply give them another copy. In this way you do not waste a lot of time developing home programs that won't be used. When the strategies are applied and found to be helpful, you can then add a couple more onto the copied form and mark the current date on it.

The FAB Strategies curriculum is integrated into the client's daily educational, clinic, leisure, and family routines. Strategies do not need to be implemented a specific number of times, so families are not set up to feel guilty if they don't perform a pre-specified number of strategies, and the strategies are embedded in the client's daily routine. However, strategies that are recommended very often can be useful for specific staff (such as when a client has one or two staff members consistently assigned to him to provide safety and behavioral support). Functional behavioral goals are developed in conjunction with the client, family, and other team members, and baseline data are gathered. After two weeks of regularly using the FAB Strategies, the client's goal progress is objectively reassessed through a comparison of the current goal data and the initial baseline data.

On the basis of this comparison, the team continues, modifies, or discontinues the individualized FAB Strategies. Goals can be revised, new baseline data gathered, and the new date and revisions noted on the FAB Strategies form. Every team member should be given the current version of the FAB Strategies form in order to encourage coordination of the program across disciplines. The form should be copied and dated before being distributed for use in home programs.

Choosing Strategies from the FAB Strategies Form

When selecting individual FAB Strategies for students with complex behavioral challenges, it is important that all the significant developmental, mental health, and sensory challenges contributing to the problem be assessed. It is also important to consider the client's chronological age and developmental age in each area of functioning, current environment and services, and future needs. Many individuals with complex behavior challenges were not provided with typical age-appropriate developmental experiences (e.g., using swings), making them useful activities. My typically developing fourteen-year-old son is no longer interested in using suspended swings because as a young child he integrated the sensory experiences provided by swings. In contrast, I work with many teenagers who are academically on or above grade level who are motivated to use suspended swings because they did not process the sensory experiences of movement through swinging when they were younger.

Specific developmental disabilities frequently contribute to complex behavior challenges; these include intellectual disabilities, cerebral palsy, and autism spectrum disorders. In addition to a client's chronological age, it is important to consider their developmental age in all areas (social-emotional, cognitive, academic, gross motor, fine motor, receptive language, expressive language).

INDIVIDUALIZING INTERVENTION WITH THE FAB STRATEGIES FORM

Many students' chronological age and developmental age vary greatly in distinct areas. For example, a preschool classroom may include students with a six-month developmental level and others with a twelve-year developmental level, because some have significant developmental disabilities whereas others are intellectually gifted. It is important for teachers and therapists to consider the student's distinct developmental age and their chronological age to determine the equipment and activities that will best motivate the student and promote learning.

Significant mental health problems can be caused by post-traumatic stress, oppositional defiant, intermittent explosive, anxiety, depressive, bipolar, substance abuse, and borderline personality disorders. Sensory processing challenges are distinct from, but more commonly occur in conjunction with, developmental and mental health disorders and distinctly interfere with functional behavioral skills. The sensory behavioral strategies curriculum addresses these interrelated behavioral, developmental, and mental health challenges through coordinated intervention by parents, teachers, physicians, nurses, and occupational, physical, speech/language, and mental health therapists.

Because of the distinct needs of preschool and kindergarten students and teachers, I developed an alternative version of the FAB Strategies form, called the FAB Strategies Pre-K & Kindergarten form. Strategies that are unique to this form were designated in italics in the preceding chapters. Procedures for using the FAB Strategies Pre-K & Kindergarten form are the same as those for using the FAB Strategies form, but it gives more strategies that preschool and kindergarten classroom teachers can apply, because students with complex behavioral challenges at that age are often not yet identified as having special needs or given therapy services (see Figure 6.2).

At discharge, all the strategies that have helped improve behavior are listed using the FAB Strategies Form Template (available at www.fabstrategies.org). Unlike the previously mentioned hand-checked FAB Strategies form programs used for consultation, the template provides a comprehensive list of the strategies for use with a particular student. The FAB Strategies Form Template is a Word document that can be emailed to the student's parents as well as subsequent therapists and teachers. The therapist's email address is also included, should future teachers and therapists want to contact them. A printout of this template is also included in the student's school and hospital records.

Figures 6.3 through 6.8 provide six examples of individualized FAB Strategies form programs that were developed, with all identifying information deleted. Figure 6.3 is the FAB Strategies program for a thirteen-year-old student with Autism Spectrum Disorder, Oppositional Defiant Disorder, and typical intelligence. A variety of strategies are integrated to reduce his head banging behavior.

The head crown and other touch strategies are used to safely provide sensory input similar to the input he is receiving from head banging. Other positive behavioral support strategies include: having him ask permission to kid with others, providing breaks, offering preferred tasks, and interspersing learned tasks (in which he is given five new math problems instead of ten, so every other problem is one he knows and can be reinforced for completing successfully). A behavioral strategy developed

FAB FUNCTIONALLY ALERT BEHAVIOR STRATEGIES

for this student that appeared extremely helpful was for the therapist or teacher to leave the room if he begins yelling or acting rude.

Figure 6.4A is the FAB Strategies form for a fourteen-year-old with severe Intellectual and Autism Spectrum Disorder as well as Sensory Sensitivity who aggressively slapped therapists and teachers for no apparent reason. Based on results from the Sensory Profile, Questions About Behavior Function (see Figure 6.4B), and preference assessment, specific strategies were developed. Strategies focused on giving the boy a non-aggressive way to ask for attention, request to get out of tasks, and manage high arousal levels. It was determined that individual attention, yogurt, sherbet, and music were extremely effective reinforcers. To manage his arousal level and reduce aggression triggers, staff was directed to remove their phones and glasses, use slow speech and pacing, and avoid and lower demands when the student was in a stimulating environment.

Figure 6.5 presents a different FAB Strategies form for a fourteen-year-old with severe intellectual disability and aggression as well as significantly increased tactile sensitivity and auditory filtering difficulties. A visual schedule, preparing and limiting transitions, as well as many touch and movement activities are included to reduce her physical aggression.

Figure 6.6 is the FAB Strategies form for a sixteen-year-old with drug abuse and psychosis. The form provides strategies that can be used by occupational, physical, and speech therapists as well as teachers who work with adolescents with behavioral challenges. Initially weightlifting and cardio exercise were used as motivating calming activities, and gradually touch strategies were added to redirect the student from auditory hallucinations.

Figures 6.7 and 6.8 are the FAB Strategies form for two teens with a history of sexual abuse who engaged in self-injurious behavior. These diagrams provide useful strategies for therapists and teachers working with adolescents who have a history of sexual abuse. In responding to their preferences, the student in Figure 6.7 utilized touch strategies, while no touch strategies were used for the student in Figure 6.8. Both students benefited from the strategy to decrease, then if needed, gradually increase sensory input so a quiet alert state could be achieved. Also, both were taught about their sensory modulation differences, to monitor their arousal levels, offered use of a sensory coping area, given access to fidget toys, and reinforced for attempts to use self-brushing to decrease their self-injurious behaviors.

INDIVIDUALIZING INTERVENTION WITH THE FAB STRATEGIES FORM

Figure 6.2 FAB STRATEGIES PRE-K & KINDERGARTEN FORM

Copyright © 2019 by John Pagano, Ph.D., OTR/L, www.fabstrategies.org

X: therapist   √: family/teacher   A: Attachment

Student: _____ Date(s): _____
Teacher/Therapist: _____ Contact: _____
Goals: _____

A. ENVIRONMENTAL ADAPTATION
____ **Weighted-Blanket-Vest-Pressure-Shorts/Pencil grip/Clip-Slant board/Chewy/Ear press**
____ Sit: Stable-Separate-Near teacher-Carrel-Disk-Therapy ball on a cradle/Headphones
____ Prepare-Limit Transitions/Trays/Carpet square/Fidgets/Comfort Box-Bag/Sensory coping area
____ Visual: List-Picture Schedule-If then/Decrease, then if needed gradually increase sensory input
____ Choosing 1 activity from . . . 4 choices; do ___ minutes minimum; clean up before next task

B. SENSORY MODULATION
____ Arousal level-Color-Scent/Anger meter/Feeling wheel/Feelings vs. behavior/Coping strategies
____ Circles: Neck-Shoulders-Hips/Tense & relax/Breathing: Hand-Bird/Mindful clock: Sitting-Standing
____ Wall: Press-Push-ups-Marine/Deliver: Message-Box/Kindness/Body scan/Hokey pokey
____ Beans & Rice/Theraplast/Sand/Water/Play-Doh/Glue/Shaving cream/Rolling to Read-Math/X/Spine walk
____ Touch vibration: Back-Arms-Body/Head crown-Shoulders Squeeze-Press/Spine roll
____ **Roll therapy ball-Core/Back tech: Tap-Press/Supported sitting therapy ball-Mindful clock**

C. POSITIVE BEHAVIOR SUPPORT
____ Freeze: Shake-Dance/Red Light/Giant steps/Simon says/Social role-playing/Bully proof
____ Character comic/Coping card/Desensitization/Sensory matching/Sensory coaching
____ FAB Turtle/Priming/Breaks/Ask permission to kid-Touch/Intersperse learned/Social role-playing
____ Play Plan-Review/Scaffolding writing/Pre-correction/Redirection/Mand-Break/Tolerance for delay
____ Reinforce: Attempt-Specific praise-Point chart-Tangible-Conditioned calm recall

D. PHYSICAL SELF-REGULATION
____ Playground structure/Exercise band activities/Beanbag pass/Jump on a mini-trampoline
____ Prone on therapy ball: Hands rock-Wheelbarrow walk/Ball: Wall-Quadruped pass-Roll therapy ball
____ Diagonal-X-Infinity-Symmetry/Both-One hand-Same side knee-Opposite side knee
____ **Crash pad/Mat sandwich/Scooter Push-Pull-Down ramp/Therapy ball activities**
____ **Suspended Swing: Forward & back-Vertical-Lateral-Spin**
____ Activity: _____
____ Activity: _____

www.fabstrategies.org   www.challengingbehavior.org   www.spdfoundation.net   www.qsti.org

References: Domitrovich et al., 2013; LaVigna & Willis, 2012; Laugeson, 2014; Stahmer et al., 2011

Parent/Guardian Signature Supporting Program: _____

FAB FUNCTIONALLY ALERT BEHAVIOR STRATEGIES

Figure 6.3 FAB Strategies to Improve Self-Control Form

Copyright © 2019 by John Pagano, Ph.D., OTR/L, www.fabstrategies.org

Client: *Behavior & Autism Spectrum Disorder (typical cognition), Oppositional Defiant & Reactive Attachment Disorder*; 13 years 4 months old; SP Definite Diff More: Low Registration & Sensory Seeking; QABF found head banging primary function nonsocial (automatic, sensory)

Functional Goals: Reduce self-injurious head banging on floor to once daily or less

A. ENVIRONMENTAL ADAPTATION
Sensory coping area/Prepare-Limit-Transitions/Low noise/Headphones/Fidget-Comfort Box
Weighted blanket/Pressure vest/Body sock/Study carrel
Visual: List of activities, check off when completed/Seat near teacher/Calm face/Slow: Speech-Pace
Choice of 1 activity from . . . 4 choices; do 8 minutes minimum; clean up before next activity

B. SENSORY MODULATION
Energy level-Colors-Scents-Modulate/Triggers: Event-Body/Coping strategies
Decrease sensory input/Increase: Structure-Response time
Beans & Rice-Theraputty-Play-Doh/Squeeze through tunnel
Touch vibration: Back-Arms/Thumper/Head Crown/Shoulders Press/Shoulder Squeeze
Steamroller Deluxe up to 10 minutes continuously supervised/Roll therapy ball-Core
Back tech: Tap-Press/Supported 3-D Sit on therapy ball move: Up & down-Sides-Diagonally back

C. POSITIVE BEHAVIOR SUPPORT
Ask permission to kid/Breaks: Music-Movement/Choices/Preferred tasks/Intersperse learned tasks
Prompts: Verbal-Visual/Desensitization/Redirection to a favorite activity/Leave if begins yelling or is rude
Reinforce: Attempts-Appropriate-Individual attention-Sensory matching-Point chart-Tangible
Switch hands toss: Favorites-Coping-Guess the feeling-I Feel/Bully proof

D. PHYSICAL SELF-REGULATION
Walk/Scooter/Swim/Basketball/Jump on a mini-trampoline/Jump-O-Lina/Bat ball/Bounce activities
Exercise band activities/Punch heavy bag/Balance beam: Fwd & Bck-Sideways
Prone on therapy ball: Hands rock/Wheelbarrow walk/Medicine ball catch
Crash Pad/Scooter board: Pull-Push/Suspended Swing: Forward-Back-Lateral-Throw to target

www.fabstrategies.org www.challengingbehavior.org www.spdstar.org

References: Domitrovich et al., 2013; Koester, 2012; LaVigna & Willis, 2012; Stahmer et al., 2011

Figure 6.4A FAB Strategies to Improve Self-Control Form

Copyright © 2019 by John Pagano, Ph.D., OTR/L, *www.fabstrategies.org*

Client: *Severe ASD; Sensory Sensitive & Anxiety; Severe Intellectual Disability; Repeated physical & verbal aggression* with extreme vulgar language; Definite difference in Behavioral, Sensory Avoiding, and Sensory Sensitivity; 14 years 6 months old; Autism Spectrum Disorder with Intellectual Impairment, ADHD & Bipolar Disorder; QABF found slapping done primarily for Escape & Attention

Functional Goals: Increased safe hands to 30 consecutive minutes or more (e.g., not slapping staff)

A. ENVIRONMENTAL ADAPTATION
All staff should remove phones and glasses before & approach slowly (aggression triggers)/Slow: Speech-Pace
Sensory coping area/Prepare-Limit-Transitions/Low noise/Calm face/Headphones (demonstrate on self)
Environmentally avoid & reduce demands when in stimulating environments, as they can increase aggression
Visual: List/Choice of 1 activity from 1 choice; do 2 minutes minimum; clean up before next activity

B. SENSORY MODULATION
Energy level-Colors-Scents/Triggers: Event-Body/Coping strategies
Decrease, then if needed very gradually increase, sensory input/Increase: Structure-Response time
Theraputty/Play-Doh/Sit on therapy ball move: Up & down
Touch vibration: Back/Shoulders Squeeze-Press/Roll therapy ball on-Core progression

C. POSITIVE BEHAVIOR SUPPORT
Breaks: Music-Movement/Choices/Preferred tasks/Intersperse learned tasks
Priming/Verbal-Visual Mand: Verbal break: "All done"
Pre-correction/Humor/Desensitization/Redirection to a favorite activity in a low stimulation room
Reinforce: Attempts-Appropriate-Individual attention-Sensory matching
Individual attention-Tangible favorites: yogurt, sherbet, music

D. PHYSICAL SELF-REGULATION
Walk/Basketball/Dance/Coloring with scented markers
Jump on a mini-trampoline/Foam ball: Catch, saying "1, 2, 3 go" before throwing/Sweeping the floor

http://www.autismprthelp.com/ www.challengingbehavior.org www.spdstar.org
References: Domitrovich et al., 2013; Koester, 2012; LaVigna & Willis, 2012; Stahmer et al., 2011

FAB FUNCTIONALLY ALERT BEHAVIOR STRATEGIES

Figure 6.4B Questions About Behavioral Function (QABF)

(Reprinted with permission from Johnny Matson, Ph.D.)

Handwritten notes at top: 14 yr old c̄ Intellectual, Autism Spectrum, Tourette's & Attention Deficit Hyperactivity Disorder SensProf=DefDif

Student's Name: Behavioral, Sens Senses Avoiding **Date:** 1/2/18

Behavior: Grab/swipe at staff **Respondent:** John Pagano, PhD OTR/L

QUESTIONS ABOUT BEHAVIORAL FUNCTION (QABF)

Rate how often the student demonstrates the behaviors in situations where they might occur. Be sure to rate how often each behavior occurs, not what you think a good answer would be.

X = Doesn't apply 0 = Never 1 = Rarely 2 = Some 3 = Often

Score	Number	Behavior
3	1.	Engages in the behavior to get attention.
3	2.	Engages in the behavior to escape work or learning situations.
1	3.	Engages in the behavior as a form of "self-stimulation".
0	4.	Engages in the behavior because he/she is in pain.
0	5.	Engages in the behavior to get access to items such as preferred toys, food, or beverages.
2	6.	Engages in the behavior because he/she likes to be reprimanded.
3	7.	Engages in the behavior when asked to do something (get dressed, brush teeth, work, etc).
0	8.	Engages in the behavior even if he/she thinks no one is in the room.
0	9.	Engages in the behavior more frequently when he/she is ill.
3	10.	Engages in the behavior when you take something away from him/her.
3	11.	Engages in the behavior to draw attention to himself/herself.
2	12.	Engages in the behavior when he/she does not want to do something.
2	13.	Engages in the behavior because there is nothing else to do.
0	14.	Engages in the behavior when there is something bothering him/her physically.
3	15.	Engages in the behavior when you have something that he/she wants.
3	16.	Engages in the behavior to try to get a reaction from you.
3	17.	Engages in the behavior to try to get people to leave him/her alone.
1	18.	Engages in the behavior in a highly repetitive manner, ignoring his/her surroundings.
1	19.	Engages in the behavior because he/she is physically uncomfortable.
3	20.	Engages in the behavior when a peer has something that he/she wants.
3	21.	Does he/she seem to be saying, "come see me" or "look at me" when engaging in the behavior?
3	22.	Does he/she seem to be saying, "leave me alone" or "stop asking me to do this" when engaging in the behavior?
0	23.	Does he/she seem to enjoy the behavior, even if no one is around?
0	24.	Does the behavior seem to indicate to you that he/she is not feeling well?
0	25.	Does he/she seem to be saying, "give me that (toy, food, item)" when engaging in the behavior?

(Attention)	Escape	Non-social	Physical	Tangible
1. Attention — 3	2. Escape — 3	3. Self-stim — 1	4. In pain — 0	5. Access to items — 0
6. Reprimand — 2	7. Do something — 3	8. Thinks alone — 0	9. When ill — 0	10. Takes away — 3
11. Draws — 3	12. Not do — 2	13. Nothing to do — 2	14. Physical problem — 0	15. You have — 3
16. Reaction — 3	17. Alone — 3	18. Repetitive — 1	19. Uncomfortable — 1	20. Peer has — 3
21. "Come see" — 3	22. "Leave alone" — 3	23. Enjoy by self — 0	24. Not feeling well — 0	25. "Give me that" — 0
Total: 14	**Total: 14**	**Total: 4**	**Total: 3**	**Total: 3**

Revised 4-19-01

INDIVIDUALIZING INTERVENTION WITH THE FAB STRATEGIES FORM

Figure 6.5 FAB Strategies to Improve Self-Control Form

Copyright © 2019 by John Pagano, Ph.D., OTR/L, *www.fabstrategies.org*

Client: *Severe Intellectual Disability; Physical and verbal aggression periodically worse*; 14 years 2 months old; SSP Definite difference: Auditory Filtering, Tactile Sensitivity & Visual/Auditory Sensitivity; Diagnoses Disruptive Mood Dysregulation Disorder, Developmental Delay, & Language Delays

Functional Goals: Maintain safe hands for four consecutive hour-long periods, especially during transitions

A. ENVIRONMENTAL ADAPTATION
Sensory coping area/Prepare-Limit-Transitions/Low noise/Headphones/Fidget-Comfort box
Weighted Blanket/Weighted Shawl/Pressure Vest/Chewy
Visual: Schedule/Schedule story/If then/Calm face/Slow: Speech-Pace
Choice of 1 activity from 1 or 2 choices; do 7 minutes minimum; clean up before next activity

B. SENSORY MODULATION
Energy level-Colors-Scents-Modulate (Green apple-Yellow banana-Red cherry)/Sound machine
Decrease, then if needed gradually increase, sensory input/Increase: Structure-Response time
Beans & Rice-Theraputty-Sand-Play-Doh/Bristle blocks/Dinosaur manipulative toys/Drawing/Crafts
Touch vibration: Back-Using vibrating brush & Thumper/Shoulders squeeze/Therapy ball catch
Shoulders press, Spine roll/Steamroller Deluxe/Roll therapy ball on-Core progression

C. POSITIVE BEHAVIOR SUPPORT
Breaks: Music-Movement/Choices/Preferred tasks/Intersperse learned tasks
Priming/Prompts: Verbal-Visual-Physical
Pre-correction/Humor/Desensitization/Redirection to a favorite activity
Reinforce: Attempts-Specific praise-Individual attention-Sensory matching-Point chart-Tangible

D. PHYSICAL SELF-REGULATION
Walk/Soccer/Dance/Pass a football/Playground-Structure/Cardio/Scooter
Ball: Shoot to target-Bat/Beanbag pass/Pass therapy ball/Shoot to target
Balance beam: Forward & Back-Sideways/Scooter board: pull

www.challengingbehavior.org www.spdstar.org

References: Domitrovich et al., 2013; Koester, 2012; LaVigna & Willis, 2012; Stahmer et al., 2011

FAB FUNCTIONALLY ALERT BEHAVIOR STRATEGIES

Figure 6.6 FAB Strategies to Improve Self-Control Form

Copyright © 2019 by John Pagano, Ph.D., OTR/L, *www.fabstrategies.org*

Client: *16-year-old; drug abuse since 6 years old; psychotic; court evaluation*; Conduct Disorder, Psychosis, Borderline Personality Disorder, PTSD, Marijuana abuse Dx; SSP2 Much more than others Sensory Sensitivity & Behavior; More than others Sensory Seeking & Sensory Sensitivity

Therapist: John Pagano, Ph.D., OTR/L **Contact** John.Pagano@ct.gov

Functional Goals: Improve self-control to eliminate once-daily verbal threats to harm others

A. ENVIRONMENTAL ADAPTATION
Sensory coping area/Prepare-Limit-Transitions/Low noise/Calm face/Slow: Speech/Pace

B. SENSORY MODULATION
Beans & Rice-Theraputty-Play-Doh/Sit on therapy ball move: Up & down/Tall kneeling push therapy ball
Touch vibration: Back-Thumper/Shoulders-Squeeze-Press
FAB Pressure Touch: Back-Arm/Back tech: Press/Spine roll
Steamroller Deluxe/Roll therapy ball on-Core progression/Back tech: Tap-Press

C. POSITIVE BEHAVIOR SUPPORT
Ask permission to Touch/Redirection to a favorite activity
Reinforce: Attempts-Specific praise-Individual attention-Tangible

D. PHYSICAL SELF-REGULATION
Walk/Scooter/Exercise band activities/Cardio-Weight lifting/Punch heavy bag
Prone on therapy ball: Hands rock-Wheelbarrow walk/Ball: Shoot to target-Bat
Push-ups: Marine wall-Regular/Pull-ups
Scooter board: Pull-Push

www.spdstar.org www.qsti.org

References: Domitrovich et al., 2013; Koester, 2012; LaVigna & Willis, 2012; Stahmer et al., 2011

INDIVIDUALIZING INTERVENTION WITH THE FAB STRATEGIES FORM

Figure 6.7 FAB Strategies to Improve Self-Control Form

Copyright © 2019 by John Pagano, Ph.D., OTR/L, www.fabstrategies.org

Client: *15-year-old with a diagnosis of PTSD & Depressive Disorder with Psychotic Features; Self-injurious cutting, head banging, and suicidal ideation;* Adolescent Sensory Profile Low Registration and Sensation Avoiding more than others with Similar to most people sensory Sensitivity and Sensation Seeking

Therapist: John Pagano, Ph.D., OTR/L **Contact:** John.Pagano@ct.gov

Functional Goals: Decrease self-injurious behavior to two or fewer self-cutting incidents daily

A. ENVIRONMENTAL ADAPTATION
Sensory coping area/Fidget/Coping bag/Rocking chair
Weighted vest/Weighted blanket/Chewy

B. SENSORY MODULATION
Energy level-Colors-Scents-Modulate/Triggers: Event-Body/Coping strategies
Decrease, then if needed gradually increase, sensory input/Increase: Structure-Response time
Theraputty/Self-brushing
Touch vibration: Back-Arms-Thumper/Back X/Spine crawl/Tap-Press self: Ear to palm
Head crown-Shoulders squeeze-Press/Spine roll/FAB Pressure Touch: Back/Arm compression
Roll therapy ball on-Core progression/Back tech: Press

C. POSITIVE BEHAVIOR SUPPORT
Goal-Plan-Review/Get permission before touching her/Breaks: Movement/Choices/Preferred tasks
DBT group distress tolerance activities/Prompts: Verbal-Visual-Physical/Scaffold writing/Partial sentences
Pre-correction/Humor/Desensitization/Redirection to a favorite activity
Reinforce: Attempts-Specific praise-Individual attention/I message/Bully proof

D. PHYSICAL SELF-REGULATION
Walks/Swimming/Drawing/Crafts/Shop/Cooking
Pull TheraBand: Forward-Down-Cross midline/Punch heavy bag/Therapy ball catch
Suspended Swing: Forward-Back-Lateral-Spin

www.fabstrategies.org www.challengingbehavior.org www.spdstar.org
References: Domitrovich et al., 2013; Koester, 2012; LaVigna & Willis, 2012; Stahmer et al., 2011

FAB FUNCTIONALLY ALERT BEHAVIOR STRATEGIES

Figure 6.8 FAB Strategies to Improve Self-Control Form

Copyright © 2019 by John Pagano, Ph.D., OTR/L, www.fabstrategies.org

Client: *Severe sexual abuse; Sex trafficking; No self-regulation; Extremely controlling*; 14 years old; Diagnoses of Disruptive Mood Dysregulation, Bipolar, & Post-Traumatic Stress Disorder; Sensory Profile Much more than others: Low Registration, Sensory Avoider, Behavior & Sensory Challenges; Sensory Discrimination Difficulties

Functional Goals: Decrease number of suicide attempts, physical aggression toward family, and verbal aggression

Date: 8/8/17

A. ENVIRONMENTAL ADAPTATION
Fidget/Sensory coping area/Chewy/Fidget/Coping bag
Weighted vest/Chewy

B. SENSORY MODULATION
Arousal level-Colors-Scents-Modulate/Triggers: Event-Body/Coping strategies/Open & close hands 10×
Decrease, then if needed gradually increase, sensory input/Increase: Structure-Response time
Theraputty/Self-brushing
Tap-Press self: Fingers to ear

C. POSITIVE BEHAVIOR SUPPORT
Goal-Plan-Review/Get permission before touching her/Breaks: Music-Movement/Choices/Preferred tasks
Prompts: Verbal-Visual-Physical/Scaffolded writing/Partial sentences
Pre-correction/Humor/Desensitization/Redirection to a favorite activity
Reinforce: Attempts-Specific praise-Individual attention/I message/Bully proof

D. PHYSICAL SELF-REGULATION
Walks/Drawing/Crafts/Shopping/Cooking
Suspended Swing: Forward-Back-Lateral-Spin

www.fabstrategies.org www.challengingbehavior.org www.spdstar.org
References: Domitrovich et al., 2013; Koester, 2012; LaVigna & Willis, 2012; Stahmer et al., 2011

INDIVIDUALIZING INTERVENTION WITH THE FAB STRATEGIES FORM

While often done in a classroom with many students, preschool and kindergarten intervention is particularly important because at this age, children's brains are more adaptable and behavioral habits are not yet fully engrained. Ages three through six are years when children are most developmentally ready to benefit from services, but many schools and pediatricians have not yet made them eligible to receive them.

Thus I developed the FAB Strategies Pre-K & Kindergarten form for use by teachers and parents whose children have not yet qualified for services. The FAB Strategies Pre-K & Kindergarten form also helps teachers and therapists to integrate behavior goals and strategies that improve learning across disciplines and settings for students who are receiving extensive educational services, related services, and medical intervention.

The past twenty-one years of using, modifying, and teaching the FAB Strategies curriculum has improved my collaboration with teachers and other professionals. The FAB Strategies curriculum has also increased my motivation for working with students who have complex behavioral challenges. It is my hope that using the FAB Strategies curriculum and resources promotes your effectiveness in developing individualized, multidisciplinary interventions for students with complex behavioral challenges in individual, small group, and classroom interventions.

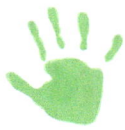

AFTERWORD

Expanding the Application of the FAB Strategies Curriculum

This book begins your journey in applying the FAB Strategies curriculum, yet many opportunities exist to expand your proficiency and application. Extensive resources are available online at www.fabstrategies.org; on Facebook at www.Facebook.com/FABStrategies; and on Pinterest at www.pinterest.com/FABStrategies/.

Many workshops are available to expand your application of the FAB Strategies program. These include a one-day workshop for preschool and kindergarten teachers and therapists, and a two-day "train the trainer" workshop that empowers teachers and school therapists to train other school professionals. An advanced two-day training is available for therapists; here you will learn advanced strategies and consult with other professionals. Finally, a four-day training is available for professionals who want to become certified FAB Strategies teachers.

Any therapists, teachers, parents, or facilities interested in individualized training, consultation, or resources are urged to contact me at JLP96007@yahoo.com.

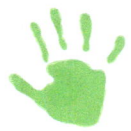

REFERENCES

Introduction

1. Ashburner JK, Rodger SA, Ziviani JM, Hinder EA. Optimizing participation of children with autism spectrum disorder experiencing sensory challenges: A clinical reasoning framework. *Can J Occup Ther.* 2014;81(1):29–38.
2. Taylor RR, Lee SW, Kielhofner G. Within the therapeutic relationship: Results from a nationwide study. *OTJR (Thorofare N J).* 2011;31(1):6.
3. Stoffel VC. From heartfelt leadership to compassionate care. *Am J Occup Ther.* 2013;67(6):633–640.
4. Pagano JL. Parental perceptions of feeding young children with developmental and eating problems [dissertation]. Storrs: University of Connecticut; 2000. AAI9988046. http://digitalcommons.uconn.edu/dissertations/AAI9988046.
5. Centering prayer [website]. Butler (NJ): Contemplative Outreach Ltd. www.centeringprayer.com.
6. Fox J, Gutierrez D, Haas J, Durnford S. (2016). Centering prayer's effects on psycho-spiritual outcomes: A pilot outcome study. *Ment Health Relig Cult.* 2016;19(4):379–392.
7. Caldwell B, Albert C, Azeem, MW, et al. Successful seclusion and restraint prevention effort in child and adolescent programs. *J Psychosoc Nurs Ment Health Serv.* 2014;52(11):30–38.
8. Pagano J. FAB (Functionally Alert Behavior) Strategies to improve self-control. March 1, 2015. http://files.eric.ed.gov/fulltext/ED555615.pdf.

Chapter 1

1. Kinnealey M, Pfeiffer B, Miller J, et al. Effect of classroom modification on attention and engagement of students with autism or dyspraxia. *Am J Occup Ther.* 2012;66:511–519.
2. Zentall SS, Tom-Wright K, Lee J. Psychostimulant and sensory stimulation interventions that target the reading and math deficits of students with ADHD. *J Atten Disord.* 2013;17(4):308–329.

3. West M, Melvin G, McNamara F, Gordon M. An evaluation of the use and efficacy of a sensory room within an adolescent psychiatric inpatient unit. *Aust Occup Ther J.* 2017;64(3):253–263.
4. Seckman A, Paun O, Heipp B, et al. Evaluation of the use of a sensory room on an adolescent inpatient unit and its impact on restraint and seclusion prevention. *J Child Adolesc Psychiatr Nurs.* 2017;30(2):90–97.
5. Shapiro M, Sgan-Cohen HD, Parush S, Melmed RN. Influence of adapted environment on the anxiety of medically treated children with developmental disability. *J Pediatr.* 2009;154(4):546–550.
6. Lin HY, Lee P, Chang WD, Hong FY. Effects of weighted vests on attention, impulse control, and on-task behavior in children with attention deficit hyperactivity disorder. *Am J Occup Ther.* 2014;68:149–158. doi: 10.5014/ajot.2014.009365.
7. Buckle F, Franzsen D, Bester J. The effect of the wearing of weighted vests on the sensory behaviour of learners diagnosed with attention deficit hyperactivity disorder within a school context. *S Afr J Occup Ther.* 2011;41(3):36–42.
8. Taylor CJ, Spriggs AD, Ault MJ, Flanagan S, Sartini EC. A systematic review of weighted vests with individuals with autism spectrum disorder. *Res Autism Spectr Disord.* 2017;37:49–60.5.
9. Hodgetts S, Magill-Evans J, Misiaszek JE. Weighted vests, stereotyped behaviors and arousal in children with autism. *J Autism Dev Disord.* 2011;41(6):805–814.
10. Rapp JT, Cook JL, McHugh C, Mann KR. Decreasing stereotypy using NCR and DRO with functionally matched stimulation: Effects on targeted and non-targeted stereotypy. *Behavior modification.* 2017;41(1):45–83.
11. Urion DK, Huff HV, Carullo MP. MRI in assessing children with learning disability, focal findings, and reduced automaticity. *Neurology.* 2015;85:604–609.
12. Green SA, Hernandez L, Tottenham N, Krasileva K, Bookheimer SY, Dapretto M. Neurobiology of sensory overresponsivity in youth with autism spectrum disorders. *JAMA Psychiatry.* 2015;72(8):778–786.
13. LaVigna GW, Willis TJ. The efficacy of positive behavioural support with the most challenging behaviour: The evidence and its implications. *J Intellect Dev Disabil.* 2012;37(3):185–195.
14. Simonsen B, Britton L, Young D. School-wide positive behavior support in an alternative school setting: A case study. *J Posit Behav Interv.* 2010;12(3):180–191.
15. Fedewa AL, Erwin HE. Stability balls and students with attention and hyperactivity concerns: Implications for on-task and in-seat behavior. *Am J Occup Ther.* 2011;6(4):393–399.
16. Brosnan J, Healy O. A review of behavioral interventions for the treatment of aggression in individuals with developmental disabilities. *Res Dev Disabil.* 2011;32(2):437–446.

REFERENCES

Chapter 2

1. Murray M, Baker PH, Murray-Slutsky C, Paris B. Strategies for supporting the sensory-based learner. *Prev Sch Fail*. 2009;53(4):245–252.
2. Simonsen B, Britton L, Young D. School-wide positive behavior support in an alternative school setting: A case study. *J Posit Behav Interv*. 2012;12(3):180–191.
3. Green SA, Hernandez L, Bookheimer SY, Dapretto M. Salience network connectivity in autism is related to brain and behavioral markers of sensory overresponsivity. *J Am Acad Child Adolesc Psychiatry*. 2016;55(7):618–626.
4. Blaustein ME, Kinniburgh KM. *Treating Traumatic Stress in Children and Adolescents*. New York: Guilford Press; 2010.
5. Van Hulle CA, Schmidt NL, Goldsmith HH. Is sensory over-responsivity distinguishable from childhood behavior problems? A phenotypic and genetic analysis. *J Child Psychol Psychiatry*. 2012;64(91):64–72.
6. Green SA, Hernandez L, Tottenham N, Krasileva K, Bookheimer SY, Dapretto M. Neurobiology of sensory overresponsivity in youth with autism spectrum disorders. *JAMA Psychiatry*. 2015;72(8):778–786.
7. Bart O, Bar-Haim Y, Weizman E, Levin M, Sadeh A, Mintz M. Balance treatment ameliorates anxiety and increases self-esteem in children with comorbid anxiety and balance disorder. *Res Dev Disabil*. 2009;30(3):486–495.
8. Watling R, Koenig K, Davies P, Schaaf R. Occupational therapy practice guidelines for children and adolescents with challenges in sensory processing and sensory integration. Bethesda, MD: AOTA Press; 2011.
9. Dunn W, Little L, Dean E, Robertson S, Evans B. The state of the science on sensory factors and their impact on daily life for children: A scoping review. *OTJR (Thorofare N J)*. 2016;36(2_Suppl):3S-26S.
10. Dunn W. *Sensory Profile 2: User's Manual*. Psych Corporation; 2014. www.sensoryprofile.com/.
11. McCall J, Derby KM, McLaughlin TF. The effects of matching sensory profile results to functional analysis and preference assessment for the home treatment of aberrant behaviors in two children with autism spectrum disorders. *Int J Engl Educ*. 2016;5(1):368–390.
12. Bobier C, Boon T, Downward M, Loomes B, Mountford H, Swadi H. Pilot investigation of the use and usefulness of a sensory modulation room in a child and adolescent psychiatric inpatient unit. *Occup Ther Ment Health*. 2015;31(4):385–401.
13. Matson JL, Vollmer TR. *User's guide: Questions About Behavioral Function (QABF)*. Baton Rouge, LA: Scientific Publishers; 1995.
14. McGinnis AA, Blakely EQ, Harvey AC, Rickards JB. The behavioral effects of a procedure used by pediatric occupational therapists. *Behav Interv*. 2013;28(1):48–57.

15. Lydon H, Healy O, Grey I. Comparison of behavioral intervention and sensory integration therapy on challenging behavior of children with autism. *Behav Interv.* 2017;32(4):297–310.
16. Kuypers, LM. The zones of regulation: A framework to foster self-regulation. *Sensory Integration Special Interest Section Quarterly.* 2013;36(4)1–4.
17. Soh DW, Skocic J, Nash K, Stevens S, Turner GR, Rovet J. Self-regulation therapy increases frontal gray matter in children with fetal alcohol spectrum disorder: Evaluation by voxel-based morphometry. *Front Hum Neurosci.* 2015;9:108.
18. Corrigan FM, Fisher JJ, Nutt DJ. Autonomic dysregulation and the window of tolerance model of the effects of complex emotional trauma. *J Psycopharmacol.* 2011;25(1):17–25.
19. Kovacs M, Lopez-Duran NL. Contextual emotion regulation therapy: A developmentally based intervention for pediatric intervention. *Child Adolesc Psychiatr Clin N Am.* 2012;21(2):327–343.
20. Blaustein ME, Kinniburgh KM. *Treating Traumatic Stress in Children and Adolescents.* New York: Guilford Press; 2010.
21. Warner E, Spinazzola J, Westcott A, Gunn C, Hodon, H. The body can change the score. *J Child Adolesc Trauma.* 2014;7(4):237–246.
22. Brown RP, Gerbarg PL, Muench F. Breathing practices for treatment of psychiatric and stress-related medical conditions. *Psychiatr Clin North Am.* 2013;36(1):121–140.
23. Flook L, Smalley S, Kitil M, et al. Effects of mindful awareness practices on executive functions in elementary school children. *J Appl Sch Psychol.* 2010;26(1):70–95.
24. Greenland SK. *The Mindful Child: How to Help Your Kid Manage Stress and Become Happier, Kinder, and More Compassionate.* New York: Simon and Schuster; 2010.
25. Felver JC, Frank JL, McEachern AD. Effectiveness, acceptability, and feasibility of the soles of the feet mindfulness-based intervention with elementary school students. *Mindfulness.* 2014;5(5):589–597.
26. Singh NN, Lancioni GE, Karazsia BT, et al. Mindfulness-based treatment of aggression in individuals with mild intellectual disabilities: A waiting list control study. *Mindfulness.* 2013;4(2):158–167.
27. Singh NN, Lancioni GE, Manikam R, Winton AS, Singh AN, Singh J, Singh AD. A mindfulness-based strategy for self-management of aggressive behavior in adolescents with autism. *Res Autism Spectr Disord.* 2011;5(3):1153–1158.
28. Ben-Sasson A, Soto TW, Heberle AE, Carter AS, Briggs-Gowan, MJ. Early and concurrent features of ADHD and sensory over-responsivity symptom clusters. *J Atten Disord.* 2017;21(10):835–845.
29. Schaaf RC, Mailloux Z. *Clinician's Guide for Implementing Ayres Sensory Integration: Promoting Participation for Children with Autism.* Bethesda, MD: AOTA Press; 2015.
30. Aronoff E, Hillyer R, Leon M. Environmental enrichment therapy for autism: Outcomes with increased access. *Neural Plast.* 2016;2016:2734915.

REFERENCES

Chapter 3

1. Yunus FW, Liu KP, Bissett M, Penkala S. Sensory-based intervention for children with behavioral problems: A systematic review. *J Autism Dev Disord.* 2015;45(11):3565–3579.
2. Benson JD, Beeman E, Smitsky D, Provident I. The deep pressure and proprioceptive technique (DPPT) versus nonspecific child-guided brushing: A case study. *J Occup Ther Sch Early Interv.* 2011;4(3–4):204–214.
3. Field TM. Massage therapy effects. *American Psychologist.* 1998;53(12):1270.
4. Silva L. *Helping Your Child with Autism: A Home Program from Chinese Medicine.* Philadelphia, PA: Guan Yin Press; 2010: 32–33.
5. Bodison SC, Parham LD. Specific sensory techniques and sensory environmental modifications for children and youth with sensory integration difficulties: A systematic review. *Am J Occup Ther.* 2018;72(1):7201190040p1–7201190040p11.
6. Silva LM, Schalock M, Gabrielsen C, Horton-Dunbar G. QST massage for 6–12 year olds with autism spectrum disorder: An extension study. Monmouth: Western Oregon University Research Institute; 2013.
7. Silva LM, Schalock M, Gabrielsen KR. About face: Evaluating and managing tactile impairment at the time of Autism diagnosis. *Autism Res Treat.* 2015;2015:612507.
8. Piravej K, Tangtrongchitr P, Parichawan C, Paothong L, Sukprasong S. Effects of Thai traditional massage on Autistic children's behavior. *J Altern Complement Med.* 2009;15(12):1355–1361.
9. Silva LM, Schalock M, Gabrielsen C. Early intervention for autism with a parent-delivered qigong massage program: A randomized controlled trial. *Am J Occup Ther.* 2011;65(5):550–559.

Chapter 4

1. Hanson JL, Chung MK, Avants BB, et al. Early stress is associated with alterations in the orbitorfrontal cortex: A tensor-based morphometry investigation of brain structure and behavioral risk. *J Neurosci.* 2010;30(22):7466–7472.
2. Kleinhans NM, Richards T, Weaver K, et al. Association between amygdala response to emotional faces and social anxiety in autism spectrum disorders. *Neuropsychologia.* 2010;48(12):3665–3670.
3. Stahmer AC, Suhrheinrich J, Reed S, Schreibman L, Bolduc C. *Classroom Pivotal Response Teaching for Children with Autism.* New York: Guilford Press; 2011.
4. Stahmer AC, Suhrheinrich J, Rieth S. A pilot examination of the adapted protocol for classroom pivotal response teaching. *J Am Acad Spec Educ.* 2016;119:139.

5. Ventola P, Yang DY, Friedman HE, et al. Heterogeneity of neural mechanisms of response to pivotal response treatment. *Brain Imaging Behav.* 2014;9(1):74–88.
6. Koegel LK, LaZebnik C. *Growing Up on the Spectrum: A Guide to Life, Love, and Learning for Teens and Young Adults with Autism and Asperger's.* New York: Penguin Books; 2009.
7. Greenland SK. *The Mindful Child: How to Help Your Kid Manage Stress and Become Happier, Kinder, and More Compassionate.* New York: Simon and Schuster; 2010.
8. Laugeson EA. *The PEERS Curriculum for School-Based Professionals: Social Skills Training for Adolescents with Autism Spectrum Disorder.* New York: Routledge; 2014.
9. Stavropoulos KKM. Using neuroscience as an outcome measure for behavioral interventions in autism spectrum disorders (ASD): A review. *Res Autism Spectr Disord.* 2017;35:62–73.
10. Dunn W, Little L, Dean E, Robertson S, Evans B. The state of the science on sensory factors and their impact on daily life for children: A scoping review. *OTJR (Thorofare N J).* 2016;36(2_Suppl):3S-26S.
11. Green SA, Hernandez L, Bookheimer SY, Dapretto M. Salience network connectivity in autism is related to brain and behavioral markers of sensory overresponsivity. *J Am Acad Child Adolesc Psychiatry.* 2016;55(7):618–626.
12. LaVigna GW, Willis TJ. The efficacy of positive behavioural support with the most challenging behaviour: The evidence and its implications. *J Intellect Dev Disabil.* 2012;37(3):185–195.
13. Keehn RHM, Lincoln AJ, Brown MZ, Chavira DA. The Coping Cat program for children with anxiety and autism spectrum disorder: A pilot randomized controlled trial. *J Autism Dev Disord.* 2013;43(1):57–67.
14. Myers D, Freeman J, Simonsen B, Sugai G. Classroom management with exceptional learners. *Teach Except Child.* 2017;49(4):223–230.
15. Domitrovich CE, Morgan NR, Moore JE, et al. One versus two years: Does length of exposure to an enhanced preschool program impact the academic functioning of disadvantaged children in kindergarten? *Early Child Res Q.* 2013;28(4):704–713.
16. Harvey P, Rathbone BH. *Dialectical Behavior Therapy for At-Risk Adolescents: A Practitioner's Guide to Treating Challenging Behavior Problems.* Oakland, CA: New Harbinger Publications; 2014.
17. Lambert JM, Bloom SE, Samaha AL, Dayton E. Serial alternative response training as intervention for target response resurgence. *Behav Interv.* 2015;32:311–325.
18. Stahmer AC, Suhrheinrich J, Reed S, Bolduc C, Schreibman L. Pivotal response teaching in the classroom setting. *Prev Sch Fail.* 2010;54(4):265–274.
19. Brosnan J, Healy O. A review of behavioral interventions for the treatment of aggression in individuals with developmental disabilities. *Res Dev Disabil.* 2011;32(2):437–446.
20. Kazdin, AE. The Kazdin method for parenting the defiant child. New York: Mariner Books; 2008.

REFERENCES

Chapter 5

1. Shobe ER. Independent and collaborative contributions of the cerebral hemispheres to emotional processing. *Front Hum Neurosci.* 2014:8:230.
2. Diamond A, Ling DS. Conclusions about interventions, programs, and approaches for improving executive functions that appear justified and those that, despite much hype, do not. *Dev Cogn Neurosci.* 2016;18:34–48.
3. Pfeiffer B, Clark GF, Arbesman M. Effectiveness of cognitive and occupation-based interventions for children with challenges in sensory processing and integration: A systematic review. *Am J Occup Ther.* 2018;72(1):7201190020p1–7201190020p9.
4. Thomas M. The effect of different movement exercises on motor abilities. *Adv Health Sci Educ Theory Pract.* 2012;2(4):172–178.
5. Mahar MT. Impact of short bouts of physical activity on attention-to-task in elementary school children. *Prev Med.* 2011;52:S60-S64.
6. Hill L, Williams JH, Aucott L, et al. Exercising attention within the classroom. *Dev Med Child Neurol.* 2010;52(10):929–934.
7. Lang R, Koegel L, Ashbaugh K, Regester A, Ence W, Smith W. Physical exercise and individuals with autism spectrum disorders: A systematic review. *Res Autism Spectr Disord.* 2010;4(4):565–576.
8. Dennison PE, Dennison GE. *Brain Gym: Teacher's Edition Revised.* Ventura, CA: Edu-Kinesthetics; 1994.
9. Bal-A-Vis-X [homepage on the internet]. www.bal-a-vis-x.com/.
10. Van Rie GL, Heflin LJ. The effect of sensory activities on correct responding for children with autism spectrum disorders. *Res Autism Spectr Disord.* 2009;3(3):783–796.

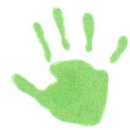

INDEX

Bold terms refer to FAB strategies listed on the FAB Strategies form. Italicized terms refer to suggested alternative strategies. Bold page numbers indicate FAB forms. The index written by Elaine Melnick.

A

aerobic exercises, 69–71
aggression
 environmental triggers, 3
 play structure strategy, 69
 redirection, in avoiding aggression, 53, 55
 reduction of through sensory strategies, xvi
 and safe hands, 42
air drawing, 71
Alert Program, and fetal alcohol syndrome, 23
anxiety disorder
 chronological vs develomental age, 82–83
 neurological habituation, 17
 and Pressure Touch strategies, 48
 reduction of through sensory strategies, xvi
arm brushing, and joint compression, 44–45
arm roll, 43, 44
arm roll activity, 43
arm shake, 44
arm traction, 44
arm wave, 43
arousal levels. *See also* triggers
 decrease/increase sensory input strategy, 32–33
 environmental triggers, and aggression, 3
 light touch, 40–41
 maintenance of as social skill, 23
 modulate arousal level strategy, 24–26
 and sensory modulation disorder, 15–18
 student awareness of, 23, 24, 80
 tapping strategies, 40
 traffic light behavior systems, 24, 25
art projects
 drawing, 31–32
 feeling wheel, 32
 rainbow goal, 59
ask permission to kid, 50–51, 60
ask permission to touch others, 50–51
Attachment, Regulation and Competency (ARC) framework, 22, 24
attention deficit hyperactivity disorder (ADHD)
 learning cues, 2–3
 weighted vest, 7–8
auditory processing disorders
 audiovisual (AV) system, 3
 distractions, reduction of, 2, 3, 6–7
 visual strategies, 10–13
autism spectrum disorder
 back tech, 46
 body-oriented movement strategies, 29–30
 and cardiovascular exercise, 69
 examples of individualized programs, 84, **87–88**
 Floortime Approach, 23
 pivotal response training (PRT), 50
 and sensory modulation disorder, 16–17
 sit separate strategy, 9
 social skills group participation, 51–53
 tactile stimulation activities, 34
 tap-press self, 41
 visual strategies, 10–13
 weighted vest, 7–8
automaticity deficit framework hypothesis, 9
Ayres Sensory Integration, 23

B

back crawl, 40–41
back rolls strategy, 70
back tech, 46

105

FAB FUNCTIONALLY ALERT BEHAVIOR STRATEGIES

balance beam, 73
basketball, 68
bat ball, 72
beanbag pass activities, 73
behaviorism, xvi
biking, 68
body awareness
  arm wave, 43
  body scan, 30
  developmental approach to, 30
  focus on palms, 29, 30
  mindful clock sit strategy, 28–29
  and sensory discrimination disorder, 17–18
  tapping strategies, 40
  touch vibration, 40
body triggers. *See* triggers
body-oriented movement strategies, 26
break mand, 61
breaks strategy, 53–54
breathing practices
  4-4-6-2 breath-counting strategy, xv, 28
  Adi Mudra, 27
  bird breathing, 27
  hand breathing strategy, 26–27
bully proof strategy, 52

C

calm face strategy, 12, 50
cardio machines, 67–68
carpet square strategy, 10
character comic strategy, 56
chewy, 8
child's pose, 70
choice of 1 activity from ... 4 choices strategy, 12–13, 16
choices strategy, 60–61
classical conditioning
  conditioned calm recall strategy, 54–55
classroom design
  halogen lighting, 2, 9
  pre-correction, 55
  sensory coping area, 3–4, 5

sensory distractions, reduction of, 2, 3, 6–7
sitting strategies, 8–10, 12
structured environment, 1–2
study carrels, 2
clinical reasoning
  in integration of strategies, 49–50
  and therapeutic intention, ix–x
  trauma-informed approach, 49–50
cognitive prompts, 62
Collaborative Problem Solving Approach, 23
comfort bag, 7
comfort box, 6
conditioned calm recall strategy, 54–55
conduct disorder
  body-oriented movement strategies, 29–30
coordination exercises, 69–71
  hand-to-knee activities, 70–71
  sequential movement, 69, 70
Coping card, 56
coping strategies
  arousal level awareness, 23, 24, 80
  body-oriented movement strategies, 26
  client-centered approach to, xv
  comfort bag, 7
  energy level modulation, 25–26, 32–34
  push-ups, 3
  sensory coping area, 3–4, 5
  weighted blanket, 7, 8
crafts, 31–32

D

dance, 68
decrease/increase sensory input strategy, 32–33
deep-pressure input, 3
  and energy level modulation, 32–34
  to lower energy, 31
push-ups, 66–67

student preferences, 46–47
suspended swing, 73–74
tall kneeling push hands, 66
deliver books, 31
deliver box, 31
deliver messages, 31
desensitization, 60
developmental disorders
  chronological vs develomental age, 82–83
  and sensory modulation disorder, 16–17
  visual strategies, 10–13
Devereux Early Childhood Assessment (DECA) program, 49
diagonal air drawing, 71
dialectical behavior therapy strategies
  suggested alternative strategies *3-Comic strategy*, 57
Down syndrome, x–xi
drawing, 31–32
drug abuse, example of individualized program, 84, **90**

E

ear press strategy, 7
egghead strategy, 41
Elbow I, 71
emotion-regulation strategies, 19, 26
energy level modulation, 24–26
  coping strategies, 32–34
  traffic light behavior systems, 25
environmental adaptation strategies, **xviii**, 1–13, 80
  adaptive equipment guidelines, 1–3
  conducted by therapist, 7–8
  FAB Sensory Coping Area Log, 4, **5**
  FAB strategies
    calm face strategy, 12, 50
    chewy, 8
    choice of 1 activity from ... 4 choices, 12–13

INDEX

comfort box, 6, 7
ear press strategy, 7
fidgets, 6
headphones, 2, 6, 7
low noise, 6
pencil grip, 8
prepare transitions, 6
pressure vest, 8
schedule story, 11–12
sensory coping area, 3–4, 5
sensory matching strategy, 8
sit carrel, 9
sit disk, 10
sit near teacher, 12
sit separate, 9
sit stable, 8–9
slow speech, 12
visual if-then, 11
visual list, 11
visual schedule, 11
weighted blanket, 7, 8
physical strategies, 6–7
as positive behavioral support, 1
sitting strategies, 8–10
structure, and self-control, 12–13
student preferences, 23–24
suggested alternative strategies
assigned seats, 10
audiovisual (AV) system, 3
carpet square strategy, 10
color highlighting print, 2–3
manipulative activities, 2–3
pressure shorts, 8
room carpeting, 6
sensory coping room, 4
sit with Theraband, 10
slant board, 9
sound-absorbing walls, 6
therapy ball within a cradle, 10
tray strategy, 10
visual strategies, 10–13
environmental triggers. *See* triggers
event triggers, 25–26

exercise band activities, 67

F

FAB Brushing, 43–44
FAB Positive Behavior Support Strategies, 49–63, **80**
 background, 49–50
 clinical reasoning approach to integration of strategies, 49–50
 dialectical behavior therapy strategies, 57–61
 FAB strategies
  ask permission to kid, 50–51, 60
  ask permission to touch others, 50–51
  break mand, 61
  breaks strategy, 53–54
  choices strategy, 60–61
  Coping card, 56
  desensitization, 60
  FAB turtle, 57–58
  humor, 60
  intersperse learned tasks, 61
  invite strategy, 51
  mand strategy, 61
  partial sentences, 60
  physical prompts, 62
  point chart, 63
  practice saying, 56
  pre-correction, 55
  preferred distractor strategy, 60
  preferred tasks, 60
  priming, 62
  prompt filter speech, 51
  redirection, 53, 55
  reinforce appropriate strategy, 62
  reinforce attempts, 62
  scaffolding writing, 60
  self-management, 53–54, 55
  social role-playing, 51–52
  tangible reinforcement, 63
  tolerance for delay, 54, 55
  verbal prompts, 62

  will like you strategy, 51
 functional communication strategies, 61–63
 interpersonal boundaries, respect for, 51
 pivotal response training (PRT), 50–57
 self-management strategies, 50–51
 and sensory-based interventions (SBIs), 49
 social skills group participation, 51–53
 suggested alternative strategies
  3-Comic strategy, 56, 57
  bully proof strategy, 52
  character comic strategy, 56, 58
  cognitive prompts, 62
  guess the feeling, 53
  I feel strategy, 53
  I message, 53
  praxis comic strategy, 56, 58, 59
  rainbow goal, 56, 59
  switch hands toss strategy, 52–53
  visual prompts, 62
FAB Pressure Touch Form, 36–39
 letter key, 36
 parental/client consent, 36
FAB Pressure Touch Strategies
 about, 35
 arm brushing, 44–45
 benefits/advantages, 41
 contraindications, 47–48
 deep-pressure input, 46–47
 developmental movements, 46
 FAB strategies
  arm roll, 43
  arm roll, 44
  arm shake, 44
  arm traction, 44
  arm wave, 43
  back crawl, 40–41
  back tech, 46
  egghead strategy, 41

FAB Brushing, 43–44
foot input strategy, 41
head crown strategy, 42
joint compression, 44
mat sandwich, 45–46
roll therapy ball on-Core progression, 46
shoulder squeeze strategy, 42–43
spine roll, 42, 43
Steamroller Deluxe, 35, 45
supported sitting on therapy ball activities, 47
tap-press self, 41
therapy ball/mindful clock strategies, 47
touch arm, 44
touch back, 44
touch vibration, 40
X Marks the Spot game, 40
goal attainment, 42
light touch, 40–41
light/deep pressure touch, 43–44
stress reduction, 35
student permission for, 47–48
suggested alternative strategies
   arm roll activity, 43
   scapula squeeze strategy, 43
tapping, 35, 40, 46–47
teacher implementation, 36–37
therapist's role, 36–37, 41–42
types of, 35
FAB Sensory Coping Area Log, 4, **5**
FAB Strategies
   functional behavior, as determinant of success, xix
   Individualized Education Plan (IEP), 77, 81, 82
   individualized interventions, and goal attainment, ix–x, 1, 22–24, 77–78
   multidisciplinary approach, xvi–xvii, xix
   sensory-based interventions (SBIs), 22–24

   workshops and resources, 95
FAB Strategies Form Template, 83
FAB Strategies Pre-K & Kindergarten form, 8, 83, **85**, 93
FAB Strategies to Improve Self-Control form, xviii, 79
   application and use of, xvi–xvii, 80–82
   choosing strategies from, 82–84
   examples of individualized programs, 83–84, **86–92**
   use of in clinical reasoning, x
FAB Trigger & Coping form, 19–20
FAB turtle, 57–58
feeling wheel, 32
fidgets, 6
fill-in-the-blank strategy, 60
finger identification test, 19
fitness strategies, 65–69
flex & extend shoulder & ankle exercises, 70
Floortime Approach, 23
focus on feet, 29–30
focus on palms, 29, 30
4-4-6-2 breath-counting strategy, xv, 28
freeze dance, 31
freeze shake, 31
frustration tolerance
   ball bounce activities, 72
   prepare transitions, 6
functional communication strategies, 61–63
functional communication training (FCT), 18
giant steps, 31
goal attainment
   in determining interventions, ix–x, 77–78
   factors in developing, 77
   Individualized Education Plan (IEP), 77, 81
   prioritization of goals, 77
   promotion of, 1
   reinforcements, 2

G
gravitational insecurity, 17
guess the feeling, 53

H
halogen lighting, 2, 9
hand breathing strategy, 26–27
hand-to-knee activities, 70–71
head crown strategy, 42
headphones, 2, 6, 7
hip circles, 27
hokey pokey, 31
humor, 60

I
I feel strategy, 53
I message, 53
I visually track, 71
increase structure/increase response time strategy, 33
Individualized Education Plan (IEP), 77, 81
infinity I, 71
intellectual disability
   body-oriented movement strategies, 29–30
   examples of individualized programs, 84, **89**
   multidisciplinary approach to, xvi
   tactile stimulation activities, 34
"Intensive Caring" (Pagano), xi, xii–xiii
intersperse learned tasks, 61
interventions
   choosing strategies from FAB Strategies form, 82–84
   determining effectiveness of, 78
   home interventions, xv, xvii, 81, 82
   individualizing assessments, ix, 1, 22–24, 77–78, 80–82
   integration of strategies, xvi–xvii
   as prevention vs reaction of inappropriate behavior, 1
   transdisciplinary approach to, xiv–xv
invite strategy, 51

INDEX

J
joint compression, 44
and **arm brushing**, 44–45

K
kidding, 50–51, 60
kindergarteners, 10
kindness, 30

L
letter ball, 72
limit transitions, 6
low registration, 16

M
mand strategy, 61
marine wall push-ups, 66
masking tape barrier, 10
massage
FAB Pressure Touch Strategies, 24
and **touch vibration**, 40
masturbation, and use of pressure shorts, 8
mat sandwich, 45–46
mechanical pressure, 35, 45
Miller Assessment for Preschoolers, 19
mindful clock sit strategy, 28–29, 31
and **supported sitting on therapy ball** activities, 47
mindfulness practice
circle exercises, 27
FAB strategies
4-4-6-2 breath-counting strategy, xv, 28
bird breathing, 27
hand breathing strategy, 26–27
prompt filter speech, 51
and physical self-regulation strategies, 69–71
stretch exercises, 27, 33
therapist self-care, xv
mini-trampoline jumping, 68–69, 73
modulate arousal level strategy, 24–26

mouthing behaviors, inappropriate
chewy replacement strategy, 8
movement FAB strategies, 71–74

N
neck circles, 27
noise levels, 2, 3, 6–7

O
occupational therapy
holistic perspective of, x, xi
integration into school culture, 66–67
and SBI strategies, 23
oppositional defiant disorder
chronological vs developmental age, 82–83
Collaborative Problem Solving Approach, 23

P
Pagano, J.
education and professional experience, xiv–xv, xvi
"Intensive Caring", xi, xii–xiii
personal experience, x–xi
parental stress, impact on children's development, xiv–xv
parents
in multidisciplinary team approach, xv, xvii, xix, 81, 82
partial sentences, 60
PEERS Curriculum, 51–53
pencil grip, 8
physical prompts, 62
physical self-regulation strategies, 80
aerobic, coordination, and mindfulness exercises, 69–71
air drawing, 71
balance activities, 73
brain function research, 70
as collaborative activities, 75
FAB strategies
ball bounce activities, 72

bat ball, 72
beanbag pass activities, 73
both hands, 70–71
cardio machines, 67–68
crash pad, 73
diagonal air drawing, 71
Elbow I, 71
exercise band activities, 67
flex & extend shoulder & ankle exercises, 70
hand opposite knee, 71
hand same-side knee, 70–71
I visually track, 71
infinity I, 71
letter ball, 72
marine wall push-ups, 66
mini-trampoline jumping, 68–69
opposite knee-*eyes up left*, 71
play structure strategy, 69
prone on therapy ball exercises, 68
pull-ups, 67
punch heavy bag, 68
push wall, 65
push-ups, 66–67
quadruped pass, 72
same-side knee-*eyes down right*, 71
scooter board, 73
spin, 74
suspended swing, 73–74
symmetry, 71
wall ball, 71–72
wall push-ups, 66
weight lift strategy, 68
wheelbarrow walk, 68
FAB Strategies to Improve Self-Control form, **xviii**
fitness strategies, 65–69
hand-to-knee activities, 70–71
movement FAB strategies, 71–74
sensory-motor strategies, 75
suggested alternative strategies
back rolls strategy, 70
balance beam, 73
basketball, 68

109

FAB FUNCTIONALLY ALERT BEHAVIOR STRATEGIES

biking, 68
child's pose, 70
dance, 68
push desk, 65
riding a scoooter, 68
shoot to target ball, 72
soccer, 68
tall kneeling push hands, 65–66
tall kneeling push therapy ball, 66
tilt board, 73
walking, 68
throw to target activities, 74
visual-motor strategies, 71–74
picture schedules, 11
pivotal response training (PRT), 49
  benefits of, 50
  reinforce attempts, 62
  self-management strategies, 50–51
play plan-review strategy, 60
point chart, 63
positive behavior support strategies. See FAB Positive Behavior Support Strategies
post-traumatic stress disorder (PTSD)
  chronological vs develomental age, 82–83
  example of individualized program, 84, **91**
  and FAB Pressure Touch strategies, 48
  mindfulness practice, 26–34
  multidisciplinary approach to, xvi
  and sensory modulation disorder, 16–17
  and sensory-based interventions (SBIs), 22–23
  sit carrel, 9
  weighted blanket, 7–8
postural stability, 9
practice saying, 56
praxis comic strategy, 56, 58, 59
pre-correction, 55

preferred distractor strategy, 60
preferred tasks, 60
prepare transitions, 6
preschoolers
  assigned seats, 10
  development of executive functions, 69
  FAB Strategies Pre-K & Kindergarten form, 83, **85**, **93**
  FAB turtle, 56–57
  Miller Assessment for Preschoolers, 19
  and pivotal response training (PRT), 50
pressure shorts, 8
pressure vest, 8
priming, 62
professional distance, xi
Promoting Alternative THinking Strategies (PATHS), 49
  turtle technique, 56–57
prompt filter speech, 51
prone on therapy ball exercises, 68
pull-ups, 67
punch heavy bag, 68
pup tents, 3
push desk, 65
push hands, tall kneeling, 65–66
push therapy ball, tall kneeling, 66
push wall, 65
push-ups, 3
push-ups, 66–67

Q

QiGong Sensory Treatment (QST), 46
quadruped pass, 72
Questions About Behavior Function (QABF) form
  example of, **88**
  self-harm, 55
  sensory assessment tool, 18, 20, 21

R

rainbow goal, 56, 59
redirection, in avoiding aggression, 53, 55

reinforce appropriate strategy, 62
reinforce attempts, 62
restraint and seclusion, xv
riding a scoooter, 68
roll therapy ball on-Core progression, 46
rolling to math, 31
rolling to read, 31
room carpeting, 6

S

scaffolding writing, 60
scapula squeeze strategy, 43
school inclusion practices, 2
scooter board, 73
scrub brushing, 35, 43–44
Second Step, 49
self-brushing, 34
self-control
  4-4-6-2 breath-counting strategy, xv
  and cardiovascular exercise, 69
  mindfulness practice, 26–34
  and positive behavioral support, 49
  suspended swing, 73–74
self-harm
  example of individualized program, 84, **91**, **92**
  punch heavy bag, 68
  and **sensory matching**, 55
  and **touch vibration**, 40
self-management, 53–54, 55
self-management strategies, 50–51
self-regulation
  Zones of Regulation program, 23
self-touch strategies, 40
  tap-press self, 41
sensory activities
  motor learning research, 24–25
sensory avoidance, 16
sensory based interventions (SBIs), 22–23
sensory coaching, 33–34
sensory coping area, 3–4, 5

INDEX

sensory coping room, 4
sensory discrimination disorder, 15–18
  effect on body awareness, 17–18
  and **touch vibration**, 40
sensory distractions
  reduction of, 2, 6–7
sensory hyper-reactivity, 16
sensory hypo-responsivity, 16
sensory integration therapy (SIT)
  and Positive Behavior Support strategies, 49
  and SBIs, 23
sensory matching, 8, 55
sensory modulation disorder, 15–18
  chronological vs develomental age, 82–83
  multidisciplinary approach to, xvi
  sit carrel, 9
  subcategories of dysfunction, 16
sensory modulation strategies, 15–34, 80
  assessments guiding sensory strategies, 18–22
  classroom integration of, 15
  communication strategies, 18
  developmental assessment, 20, 22
  emotion-regulation strategies, 19
  empowerment of students and families, 22
  FAB strategies
    hand breathing strategy, 26–27
    modulate arousal level strategy, 24–26
    self-brushing, 34
    slow speech, 12
    tactile stimulation activities, 34
  FAB Strategies to Improve Self-Control form, **xviii**
  finger identification test, 19
  introduction of, 2
  massage, 24
  mindfulness movement strategies
    body scan, 30
    deliver books, 31
    deliver box, 31
    deliver messages, 31
    focus on feet, 29–30
    focus on palms, 29, 30
    freeze dance, 31
    freeze shake, 31
    giant steps, 31
    hokey pokey, 31
    mindful clock sit strategy, 28–29, 31
    rolling to math, 31
    rolling to read, 31
    Simon says, 31
    Twister, 31
  preference assessment, 19, 20
  and Pressure Touch strategies, 48
  progressive relaxation, 28–31
  recognition of triggers, 32
  reinforcement of inappropriate behaviors, 20
  Sensory Profile, 19
  student preferences, 23–24
  suggested alternative strategies
    body triggers, 25–26
    crafts, 31–32
    decrease/increase sensory input strategy, 32–33
    drawing, 31–32
    event triggers, 25–26
    hip circles, 27
    increase structure/increase response time strategy, 33
    kindness, 30
    neck circles, 27
    sensory coaching, 33–34
    shoulder circles, 27
    stretch down, 27
    stretch front, 33
    stretch lateral, 27
    stretch rotation, 27
    stretch side, 33
    stretch up, 27
  touch strategies, 80
  traffic light behavior systems, 24, 25
Sensory Motor Arousal Regulation Treatment (SMART), 22
sensory over-responsivity
  habituation, 16
  and impulse aggression, 31
sensory oversensitivity
  learning cues, 2–3
  sitting strategies, 8–10
sensory seeking, 16
sensory under-responsivity, 16
sensory-based interventions (SBIs)
  and positive behavior support strategies, 49
  and sensory integration therapy (SIT), 23
sexual abuse
  example of individualized program, 84, **91**, **92**
shaving cream, 34
shoot to target ball, 72
shoulder circles, 27
shoulder squeeze strategy, 42–43
Simon says, 31
sitting strategies
  assigned seats, 10
  carpet square strategy, 10
  clipboard attachment, 9
  masking tape barrier, 10
  postural stability, 9
  sit carrel, 9
  sit disk, 10
  sit near teacher, 12
  sit separate, 9
  sit stable, 8–9
  sit with Theraband, 10
  slant board, 9
  supported sitting on therapy ball activities, 47
  therapy ball within a cradle, 10
  tray strategy, 10
slant board, 9
soccer, 68

111

social role-playing, 51–52
social skills group participation, 51–53
sound-absorbing walls, 6
spin, 74
spine roll, 42, 43
Steamroller Deluxe, 35, 45
sticker chart, 63
Stoffel, Ginny, x
stress
    4-4-6-2 breath-counting strategy, xv, 28
    mindfulness practice, 26–34
    parental stress, impact on children's development, xiv–xv
stretch down, 27
stretch front, 33
stretch lateral, 27
stretch rotation, 27
stretch side, 33
stretch up, 27
students/clients
    chronological vs develmental age, 82–83
    trust of therapists/teachers, x
study carrels, 2
supported sitting on therapy ball activities
    and **mindful clock** strategies, 47
suspended swing, 73–74
symmetry, 71

T

tactile defensiveness, 17
tactile stimulation activities, 34
tall kneeling push hands, 65–66
tall kneeling push therapy ball, 66
tangible reinforcement, 63
tapping, 35, 40
    student preferences, 46–47
tap-press self, 41
teachers
    adaptive equipment guidelines, 1–3
    application and use of FAB Strategies form, xvi–xvii, **xviii**

calm face strategy, 12, 50
Individualized Education Plan (IEP), 77, 81, 82
in multidisciplinary team approach, xix
and pivotal response training (PRT), 50–51
professional collaboration with sensory assessments, 18
slow speech, 12
therapeutic intention, x
Theraband activities, 67
therapeutic intention, and clinical reasoning, ix–x
therapists
    application and use of FAB Strategies form, xvi–xvii, **xviii**
    calm face strategy, 12, 50
    environmental adaptation strategies, 7–8
    holistic perspective of, x
    Individualized Education Plan (IEP), 77, 81, 82
    in multidisciplinary team approach, xix
    and pivotal response training (PRT), 50–51
    professional distance, xi
    role in individualizing interventions, x
    role in Pressure Touch strategy development, 36–37, 41–42, 48
    self-care, xv
    transdisciplinary approach, xiv–xv
Theraputty, 34
3-Comic strategy, 56, 57
throw to target activities, 74
tilt board, 73
tolerance for delay, 54, 55
touch arm, 44
touch back, 44
touch hypersensitivity
    ear press strategy, 7
    interpersonal touch, 66
    tactile defensiveness, 17

touch vibration, 40
touch vibration arms, 40
touch vibration back, 40
touch vibration body, 40
traffic light behavior systems, 24, 25
transitions
    limit transitions, 6
    to lower energy, 31
    prepare transitions, 6
    schedule story, 11–12
tray strategy, 10
triggers
    body triggers, 25–26
    environmental triggers, 3, 6, 20
    FAB Trigger & Coping form, 19–20
    recognition of, 32, 49
    transitions, 6
trust
    students trust of therapists/teachers, x
Twister, 31

V

verbal prompts, 62
vibration, 35
visual prompts, 62
visual strategies, 10–13
    distractions, reduction of, 2
    picture schedules, 11
    schedule story, 11–12
    sit carrel, 9
    visual if-then, 11
    visual list, 11
    visual schedule, 11
visual supports, and SBI strategies, 23
visual-motor strategies, 71–74

W

walking, 68
wall ball, 71–72
wall push-ups, 66
weight lift strategy, 68
weighted blanket
    benefits/contraindications, 8
    as coping strategy, 7

INDEX

weighted vest
    benefits/contraindications, 7–8
wheelbarrow walk, 68
Wilbarger Brushing Protocol, and FAB Brushing, 43–44
will like you strategy, 51

X
X Marks the Spot game, 40

Z
Zones of Regulation program, 23, 24